# YOGA COLORING BOOK

## Coloring Beginner Yoga Poses to Life with Explanations

### Gift Idea for Students, Teachers, and Instructors

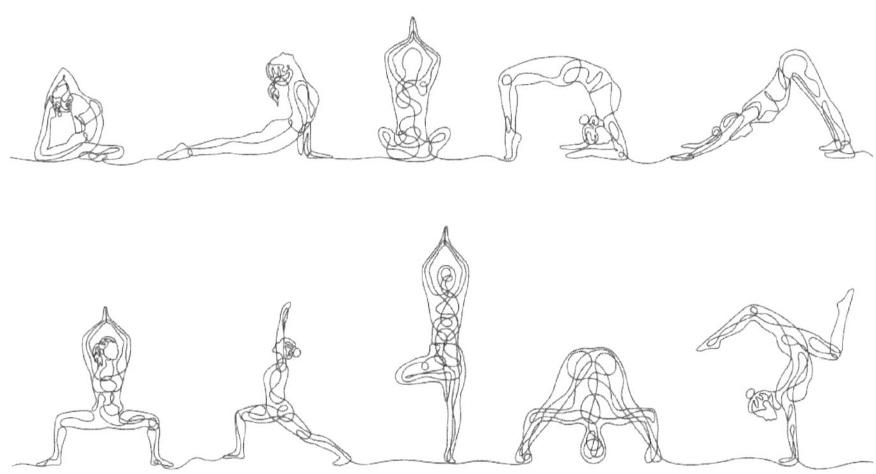

# DREAMSTORM PUBLICATIONS

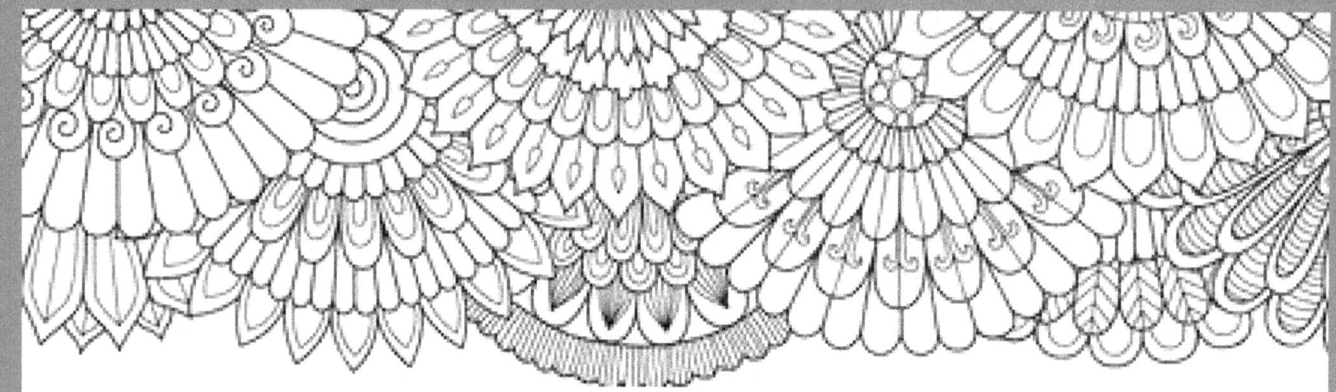

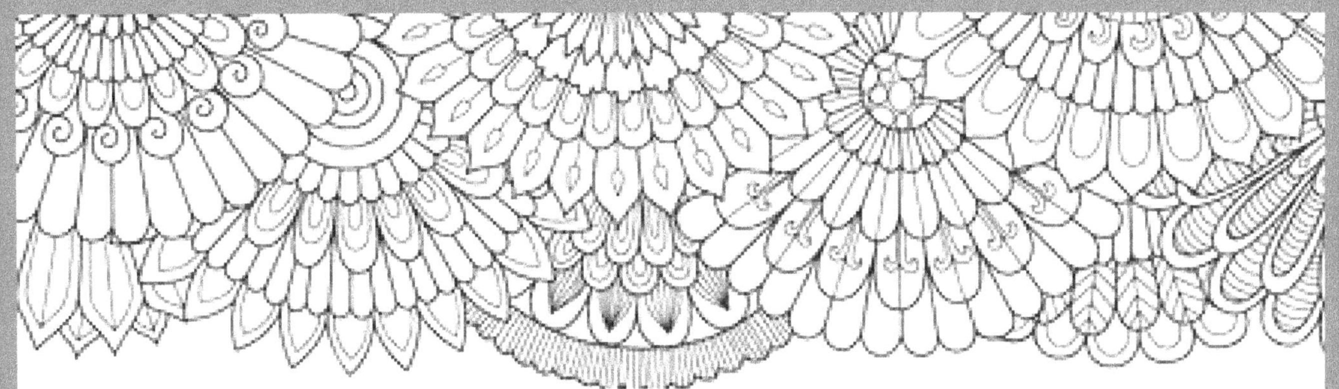

Yoga is a dance between control and surrender
between pushing and letting go – and when
to push and when to let go becomes part of
the creative process, part of an open-ended
exploration of your being.

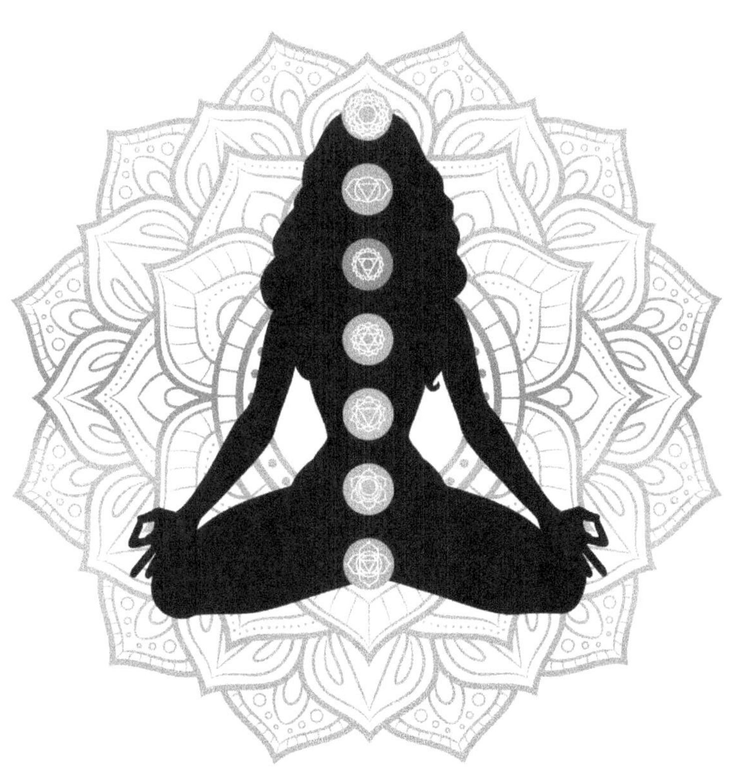

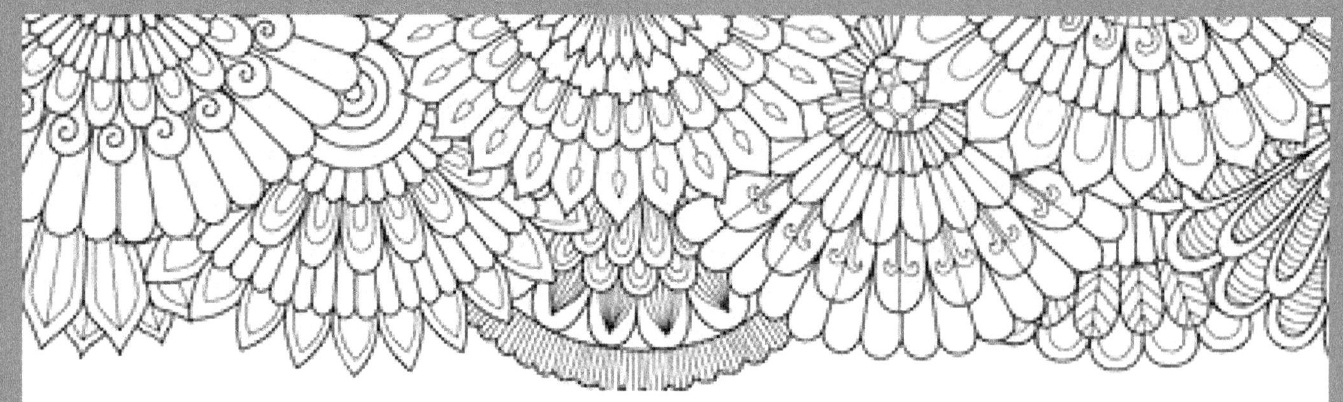

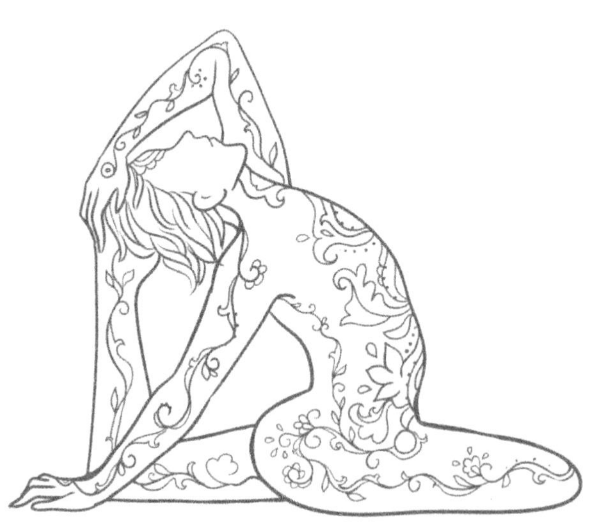

Yoga is not a work-out, it is a work-in.
And this is the point of spiritual practice;
to make us teachable; to open up our hearts
and focus our awareness so that
we can know what we already know
and be who we already are.

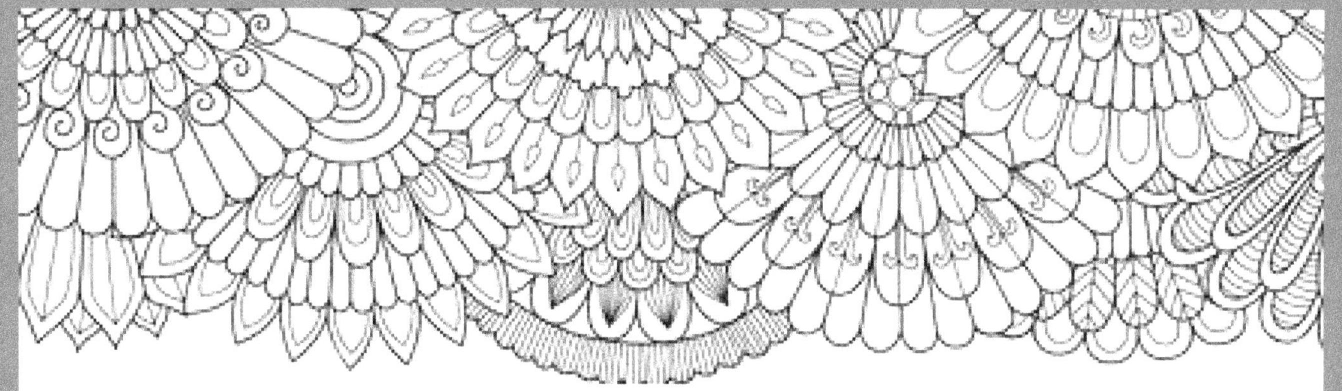

# INTRODUCTION

Yoga, which is well known for its postures and poses, is an ancient physical and spiritual discipline, and a branch of philosophy that originated in India more than 5,000 years ago. While mandalas are sacred geometric figures that represent the universe which helps you focus on doing the yoga poses. They both open the doors into your soul and get you deeper into meditation as you connect to the universe and to the highest.

Combined together *(just like in your yoga practice)*, **Yoga Coloring Book with Mandala Backgrounds,** will provide you hours of coloring enjoyment while helping you relax, remember your poses, learn new things, and stay motivated while practicing yoga.

So, grab your pencils, free your mind, and go to your favorite coloring spot because it's time to relax and unleash your creativity.

Turn to the next page and have fun coloring your way to yoga!

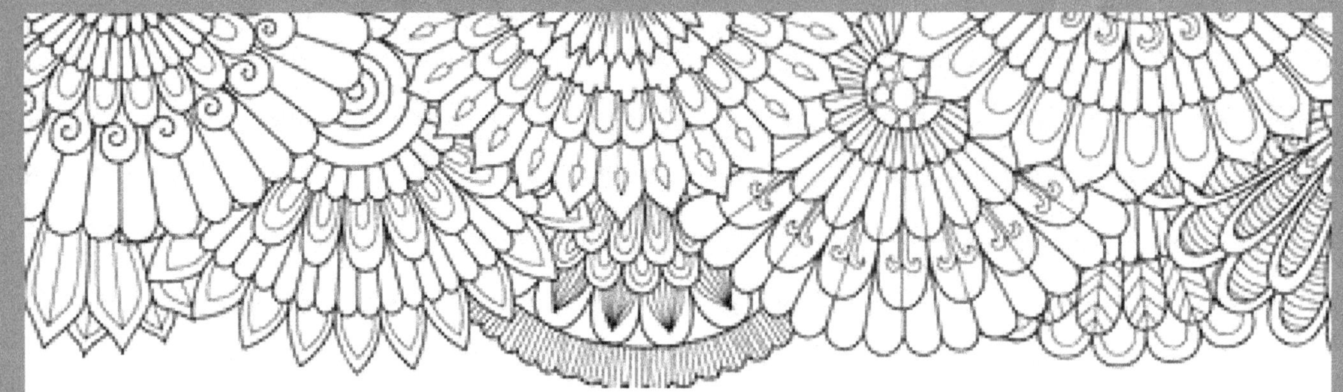

# TRIANGLE POSE

Extended Triangle Pose (Trikosnasana) is a standing yoga pose that tones the legs, reduces stress, and increases stability.

A deep stretch for the hamstrings, groins, and hips, *Trikonasana* also opens the chest and shoulders. It helps relieve lower back pain, stress, and sluggish digestion. This pose strengthens the muscles in the thighs, hips, and back, while toning the knees and ankles. It also stimulates the organs of the torso, improving metabolism. It is known to be therapeutic for anxiety, flat feet, infertility, osteoporosis, and even sciatica.

Triangle Pose can be a building block for balance and grace in all areas of your life. Practicing this pose on a regular basis will bring poise, strength, and equanimity to your everyday routine!

"Yoga does not just change the way we see things,
it transforms the person who sees."
— **B.K.S Iyengar**

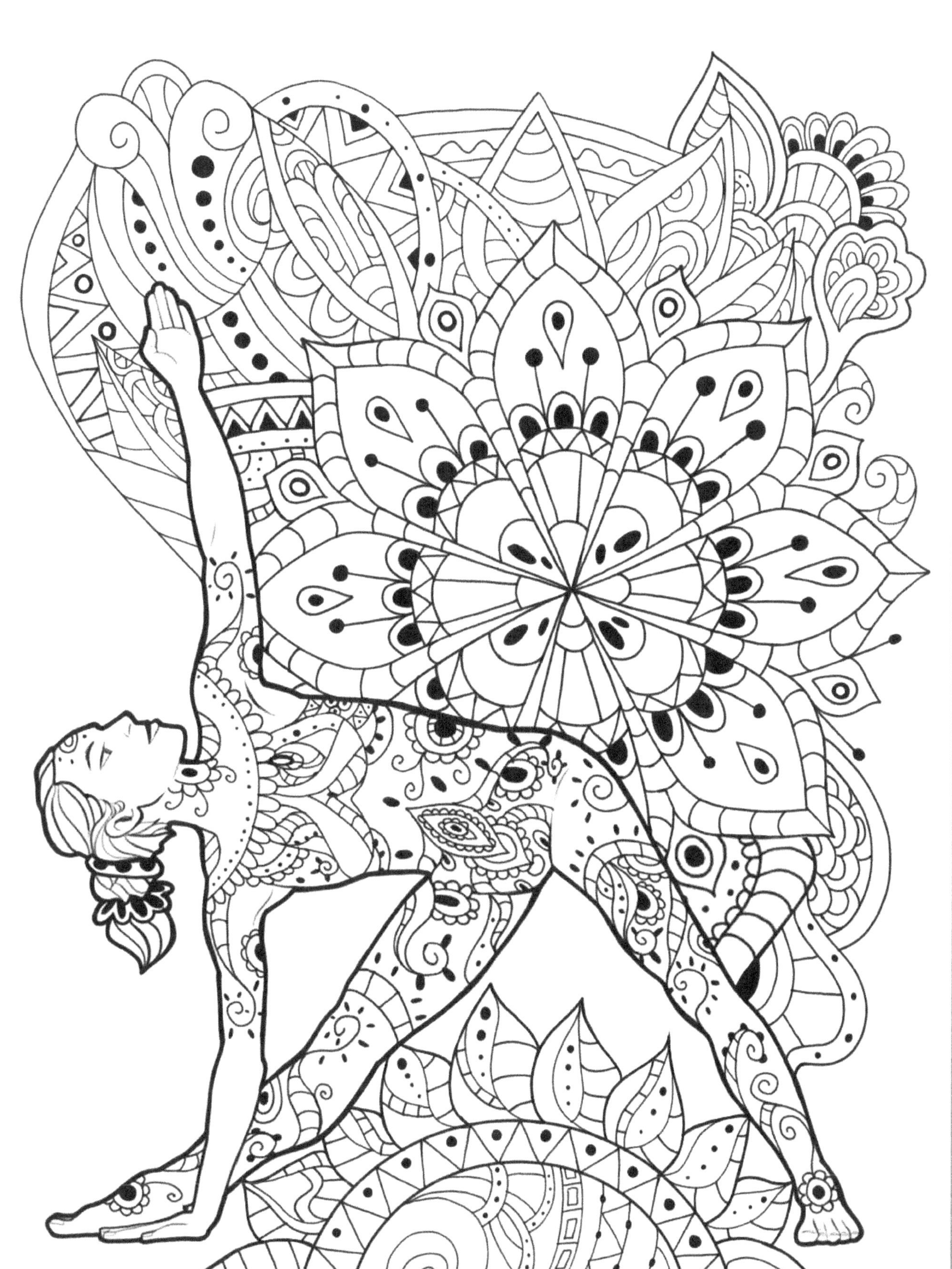

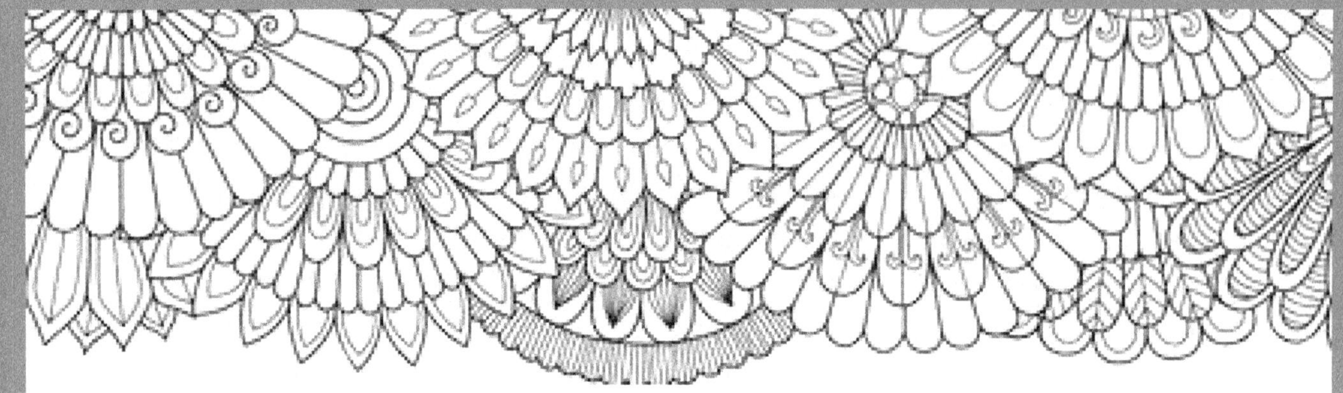

# EASY POSE

Easy Pose (Sukhasana) is the name for any comfortable, cross-legged, seated position, and one of the most basic poses used in yoga practice and meditation. Also sometimes called "Simple Cross-Legged Pose," Sukhasana is intended to be comfortable and calming.

Easy pose is a comfortable seated position for meditation. This pose opens the hips, lengthens the spine and promotes groundedness and inner calm.

Sukhasana is a simple and basic pose to come into at any time. Whenever you need to find peace, simply bring yourself to the ground and sit quietly. As you slow your breath, your mind will begin to calm down. Regularly integrate Easy Pose into your practice and into your daily life — you may notice serenity and ease flowing through all areas of your life!

"When you listen to yourself, everything comes naturally.
It comes from inside, like a kind of will to do something.
Try to be sensitive. That is yoga." — **Petri Räisänen**

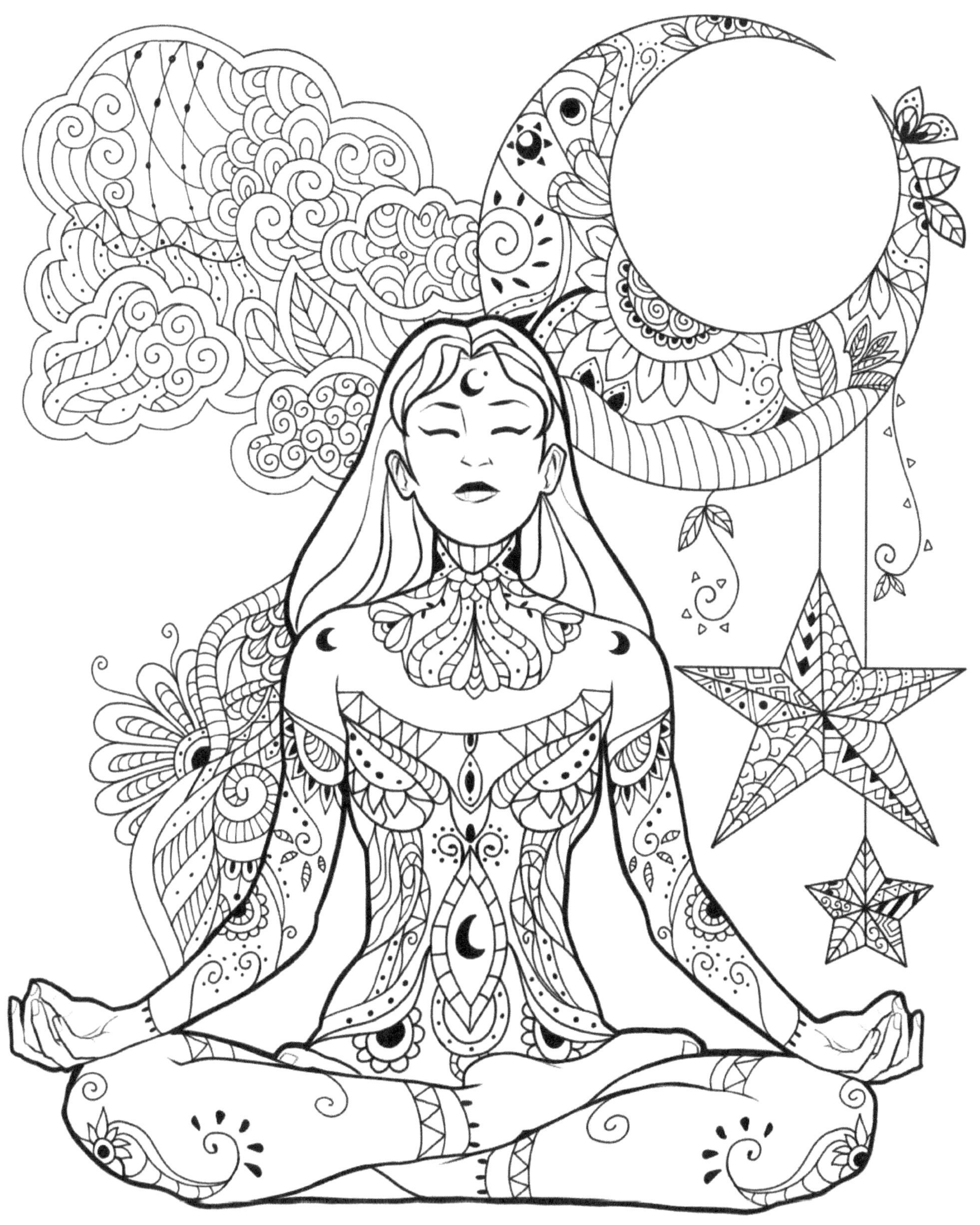

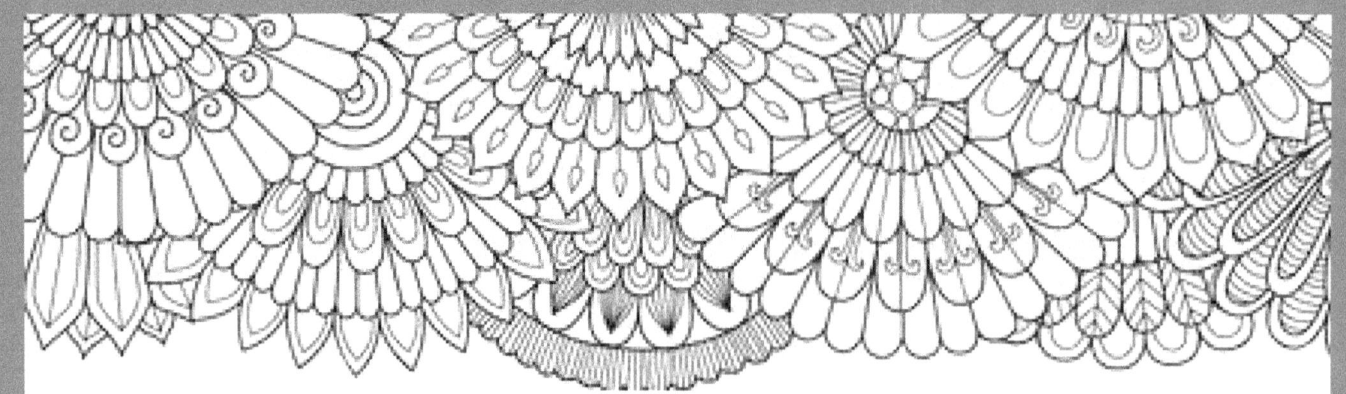

# CHILD'S POSE

Child's Pose (Balasana) is a common beginner's yoga pose. It is yoga's most important resting posture and it is a nice way to gently stretch various parts of your body. It's a chance to stop what you are doing, reassess your position, reconnect with your breath, and prepare yourself to move forward.

Child's Pose is a gentle stretch for the back, hips, thighs, and ankles. It can help relieve back pain. Regular practice of Child's Pose also teaches conscious exploration of the breath.

Child's Pose is a simple way to calm your mind, slow your breath, and restore a feeling of peace and safety. Practicing the pose before bedtime can help to release the worries of the day.

"We all wish for world peace, but world peace will never be achieved unless we first establish peace within our own minds."
— Geshe Kelsang Gyatso

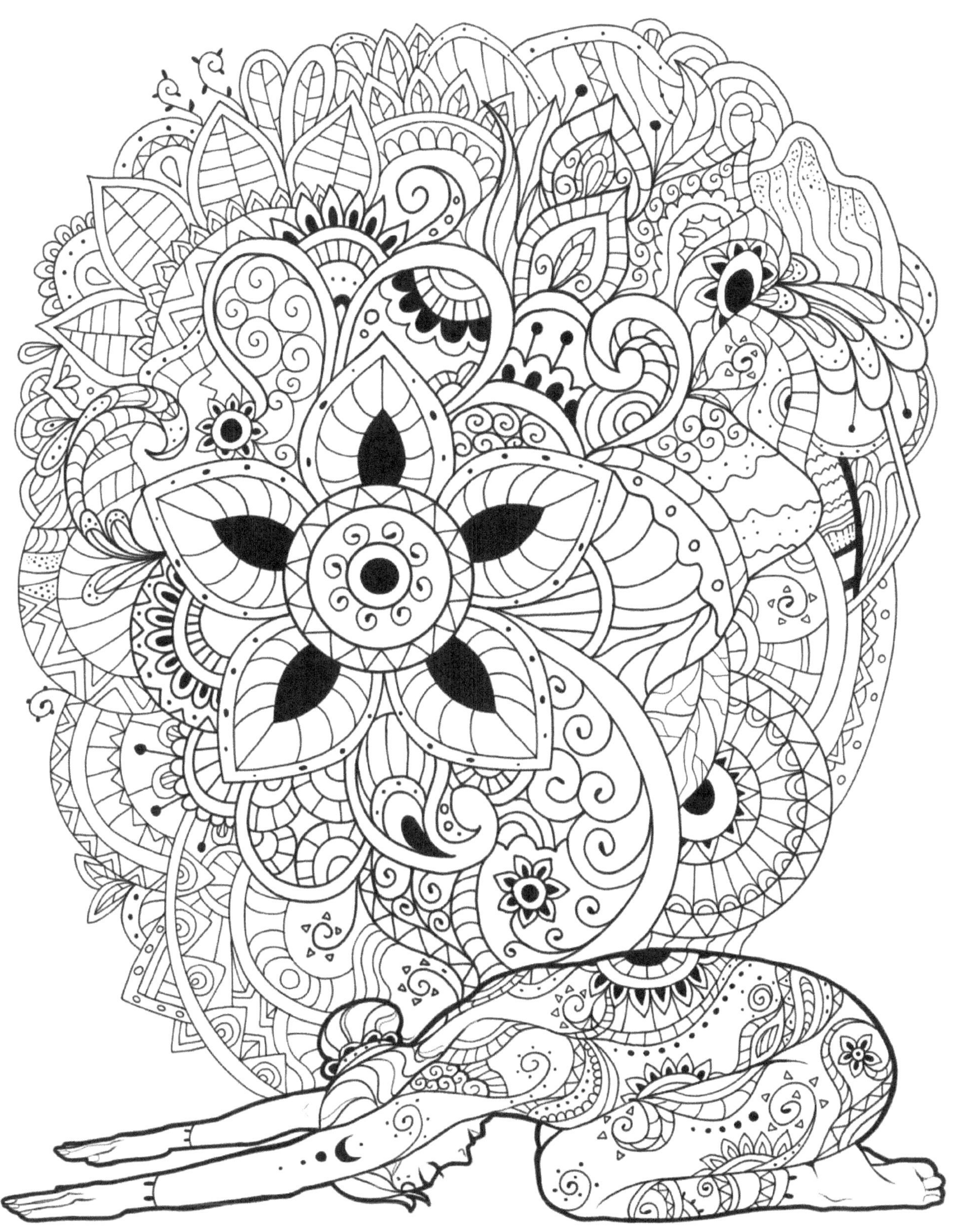

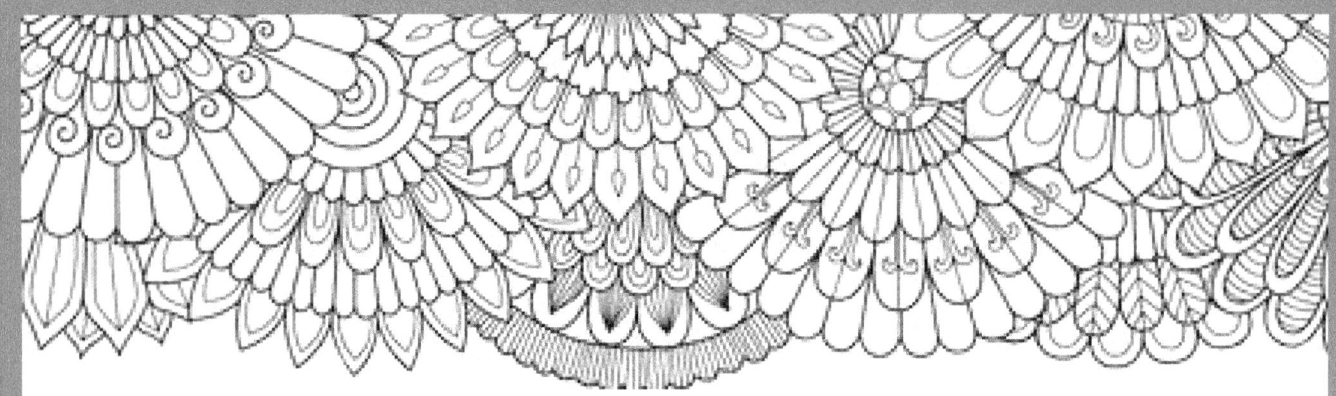

# BRIDGE POSE

Bridge Pose (Sethu Bandha Sarvangasana) is a beginning backbend that helps to open the chest and stretch the thighs.

Bridge pose builds core and lower body strength, lengthens and strengthens the spine, energizes the body, and stimulates the endocrine and nervous systems. Bridge Pose also calms the mind and is known to be therapeutic for individuals with high blood pressure.

Practicing Bridge Pose can be a potent lesson in learning to slow down and listen to your body. Your spine, shoulders, and thighs will tell you how far to take the pose. Let your Bridge be a connection between your body, mind, and spirit.

"True meditation is about being fully present
with everything that is including discomfort and challenges.
It is not an escape from life." — **Craig Hamilton**

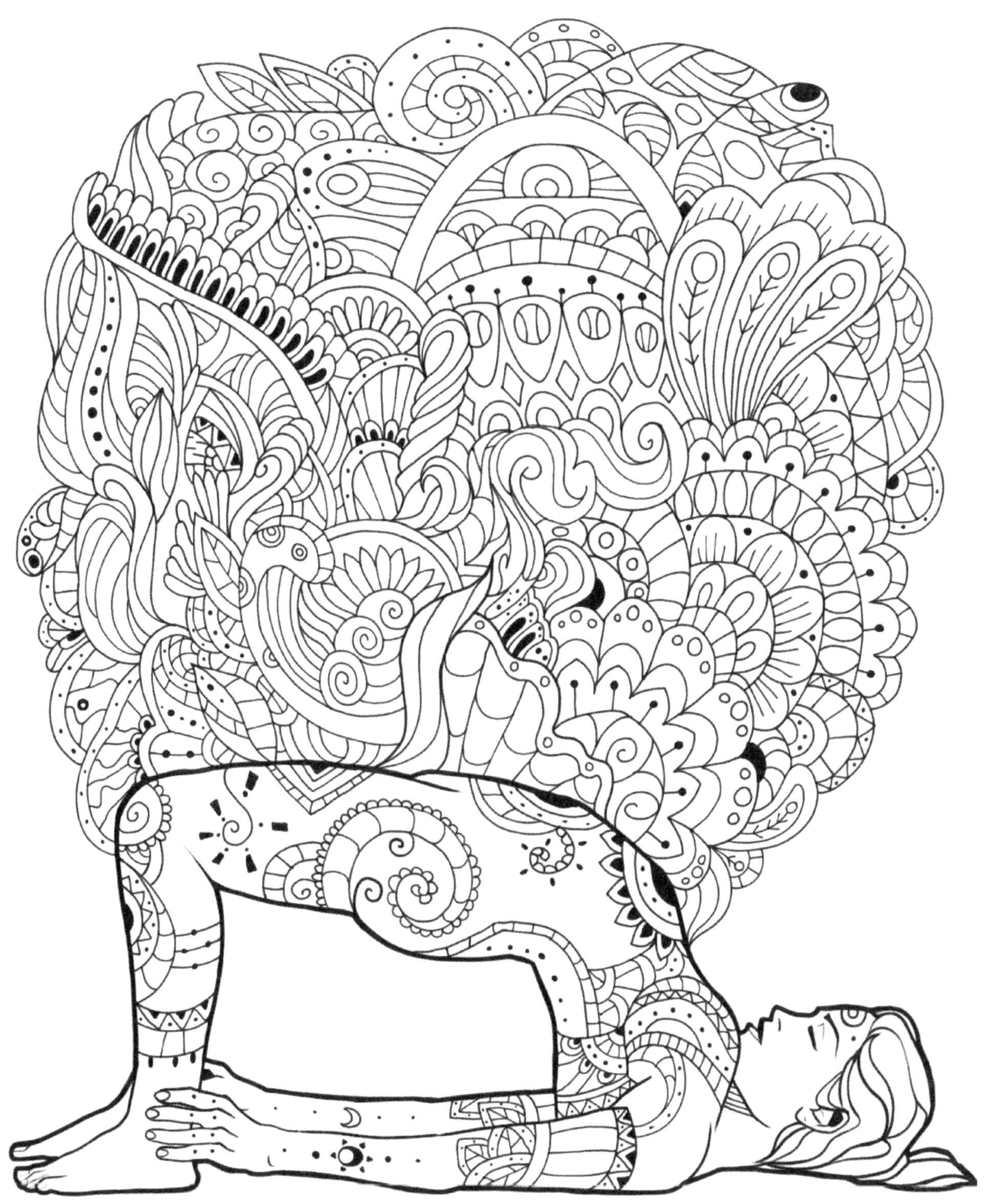

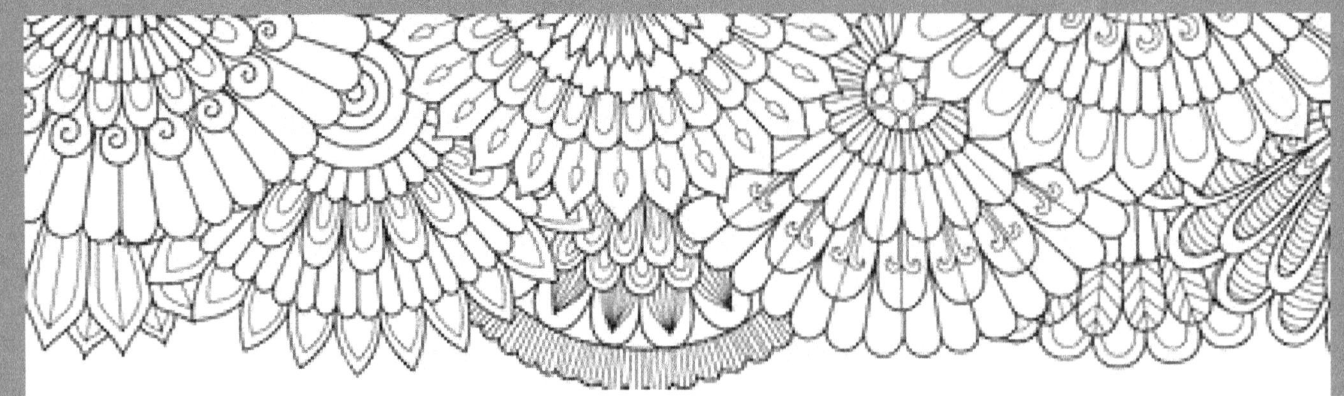

# DOLHPIN POSE

Dolphin Pose (Catur Svanasana) is a great beginning yoga pose for many reasons. It strengthens, and stretches the shoulders, upper back and legs.  It's also a pretty awesome core strengthener.

Practicing Dolphin Pose can be a great way to warm, strengthen, and stretch your whole body. It's also a great modification for those with wrist troubles. It adds variety and fun to your practice, while challenging your muscles and your mind. Vary your practice with Dolphin Pose and you might discover joy and freedom in movement.

"Yoga is a light, which once lit will never dim.
The better your practice, the brighter your flame."
— **B.K.S Iyengar**

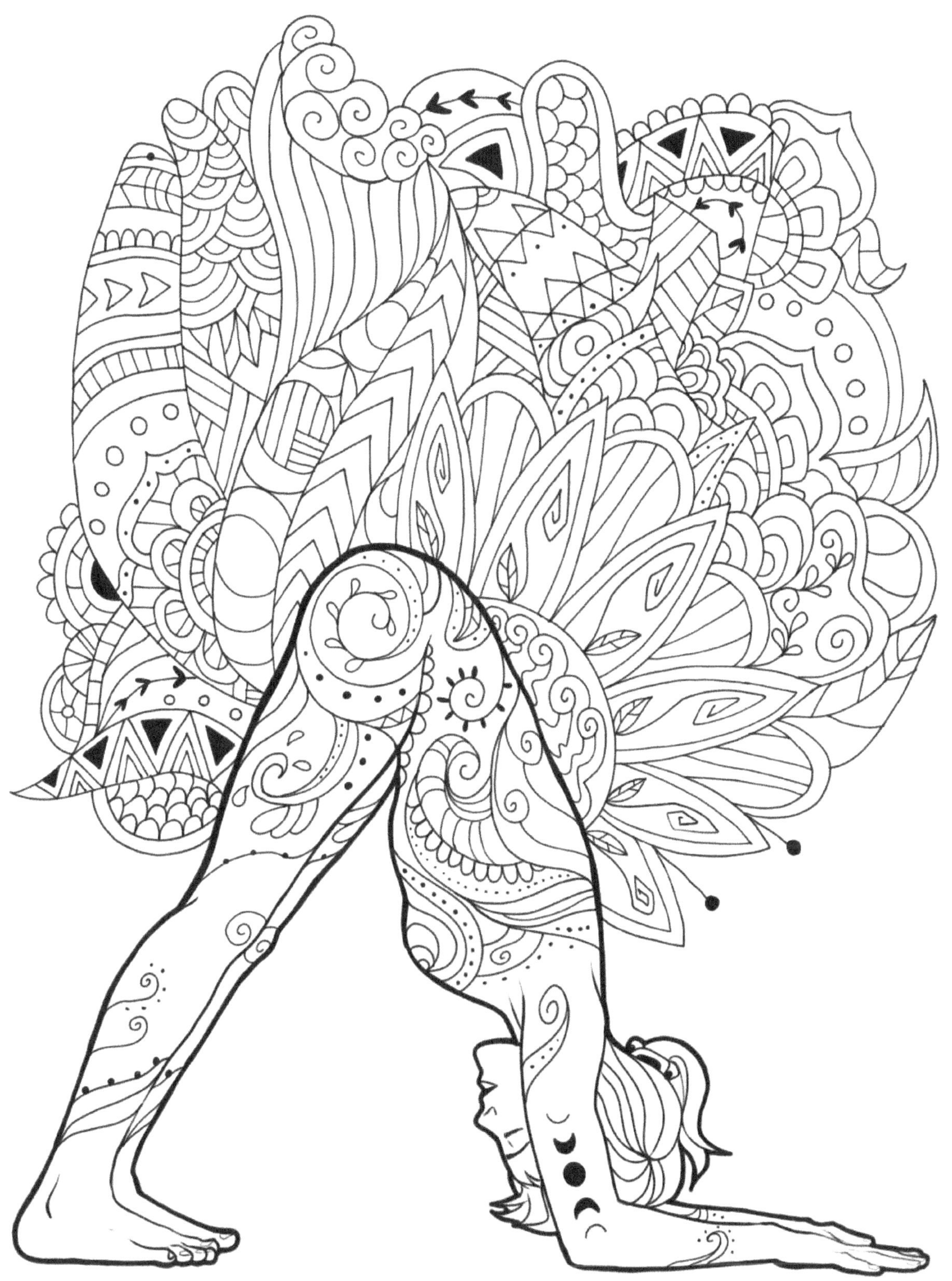

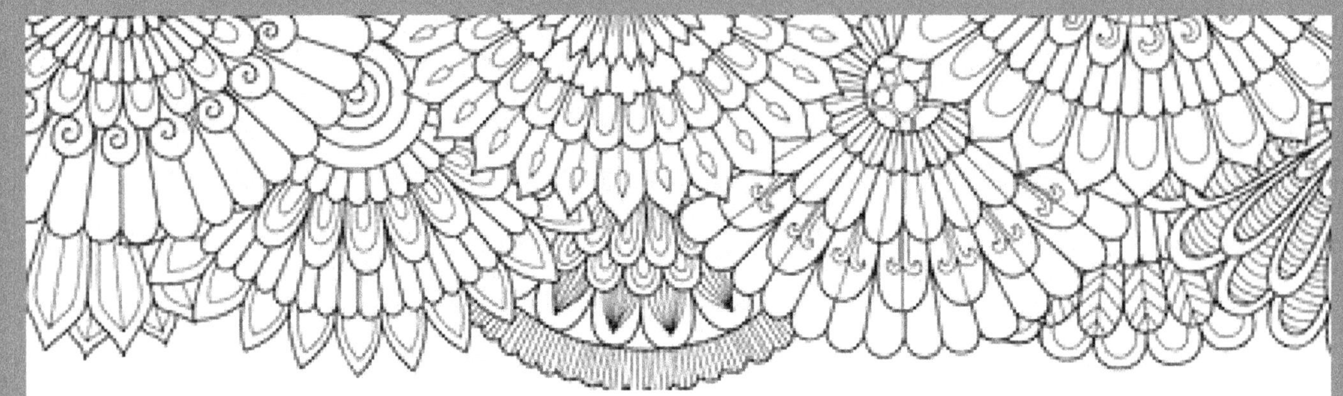

# COBRA POSE

Cobra yoga pose (Bhujangasana) is most commonly practiced as part of the basic sun salutation, also known as Sun A. Also, this is a beginning backbend in yoga that helps to prepare the body for deeper backbends.

This pose is best known for its ability to increase the flexibility of the spine.  It strengthens the back-body muscles - hamstrings, glutes, and spinal extensors. While you lengthen the spine and lift the chest, it also opens the front side of the body, chest and throat and expands the breath.

Cobra Pose can be a great way to stretch out your spine and chest throughout the day. It counteracts the slouch that comes from sitting in front of a computer or driving. Bringing more flexibility to your spine will help you to feel more balanced, while opening your chest and heart will energize and rejuvenate you throughout the day!

"Yoga is the journey of the self, through the self, to the self."
— **The Bhagavad Gita**

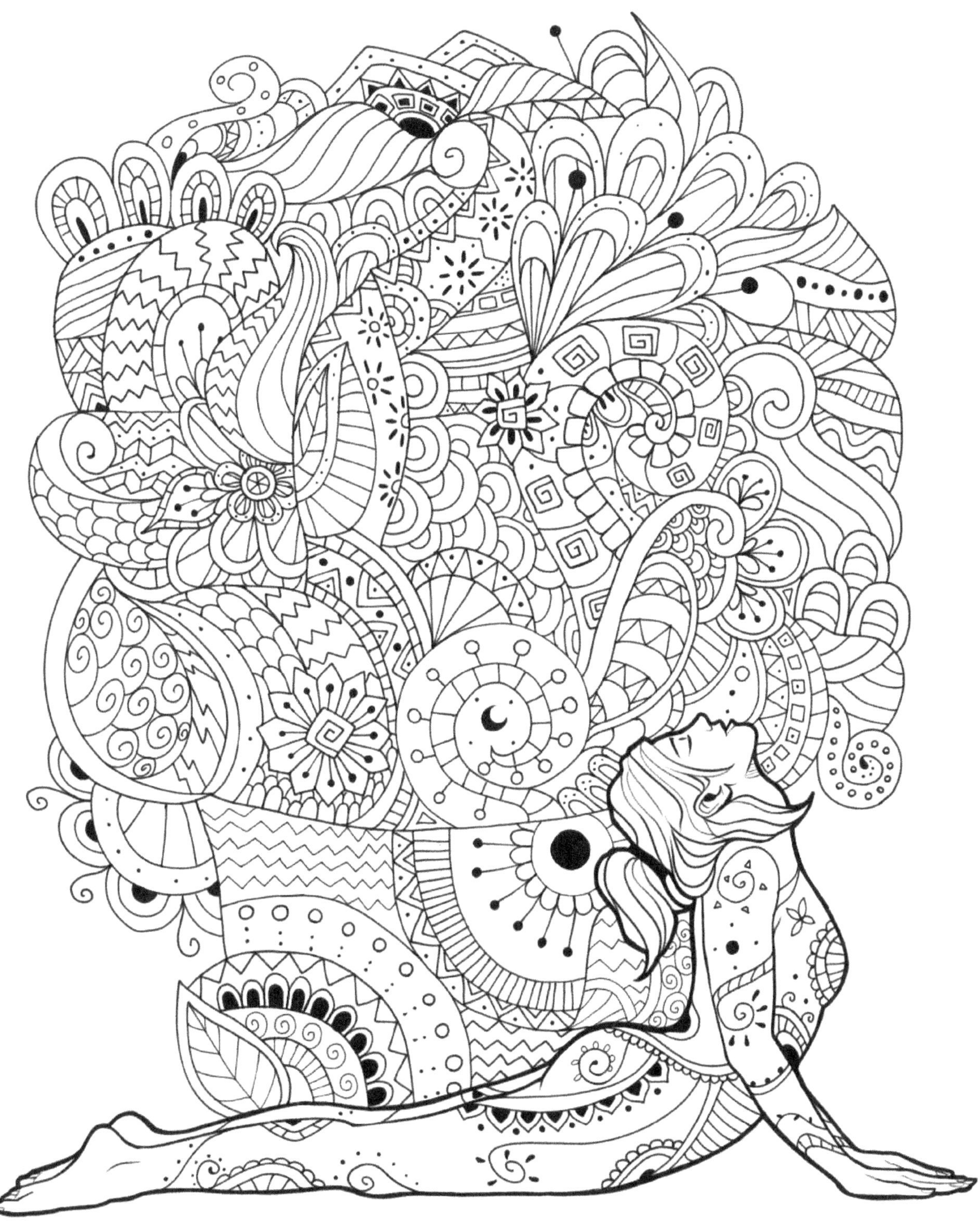

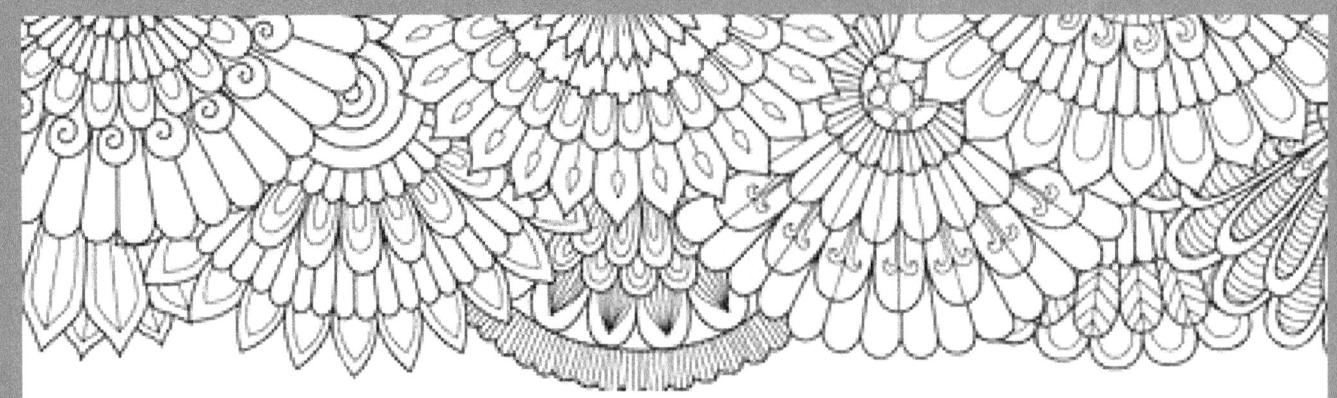

# HALF LORD OF THE FISHES POSE

Half Lord of the Fishes Pose (Ardha Matsyendrasana) is a popular seated twist. This pose invites an energy in the spine that helps to stimulate proper digestion while improving postural and body awareness.

Half Lord of the Fishes Pose stretches the side body, upper back, and neck, and improves spinal mobility. It's important to keep these areas loose and mobile to prevent pain from repetitive stress injuries. Twists such as this can also help constipation.

Including twists in your yoga practice will help you to find ease, balance, and serenity in all areas of your life. Twisting and lengthening your spine can make you feel re-energized and revitalized. Squeezing out toxins from your abdominal organs will cleanse and refresh you, inside and out. Practicing Ardha Matsyendrasana on a regular basis will keep you feeling young, vital, and healthy!

"Yoga is the fountain of youth. You're only as young as your spine is flexible." — **Bob Harper**

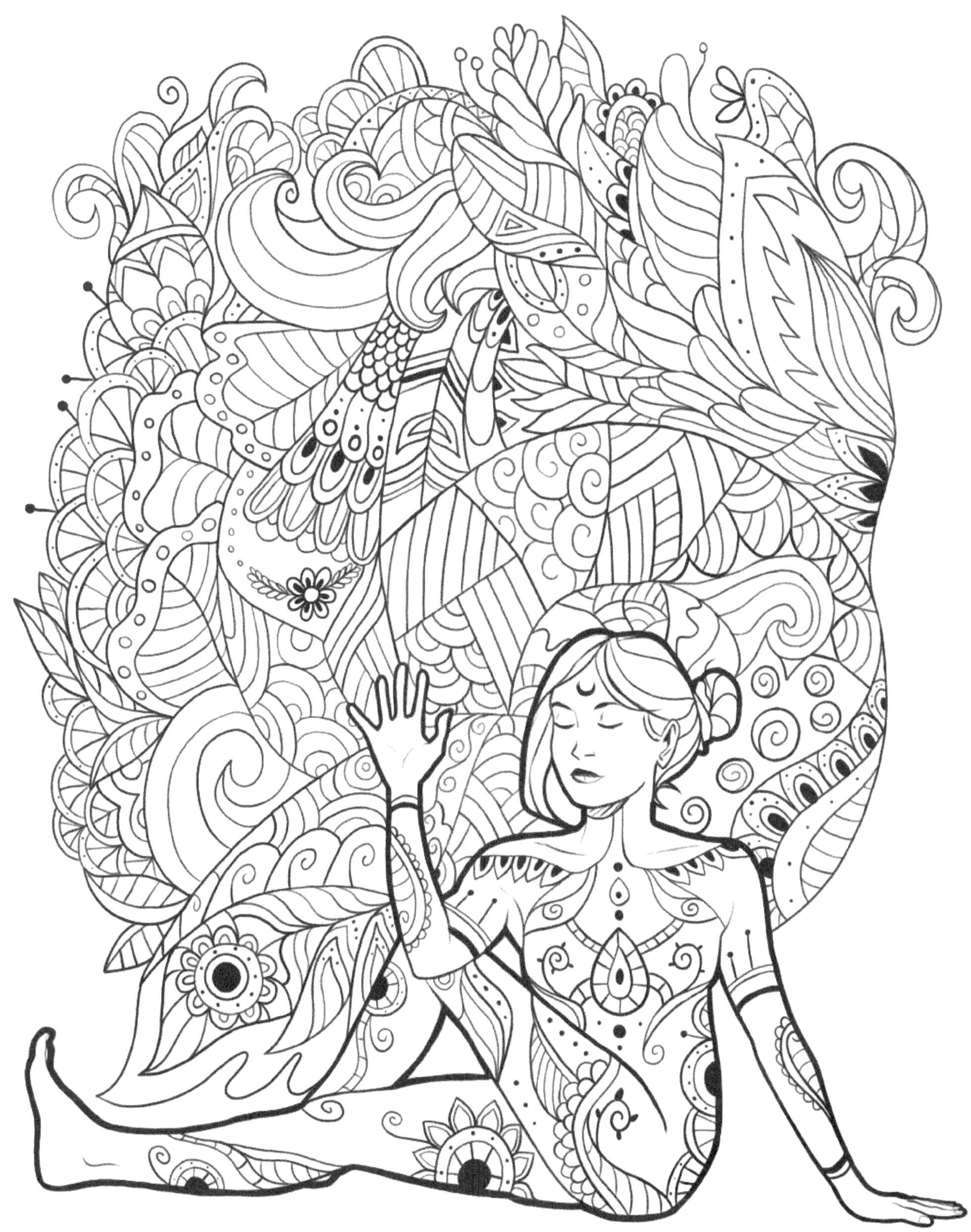

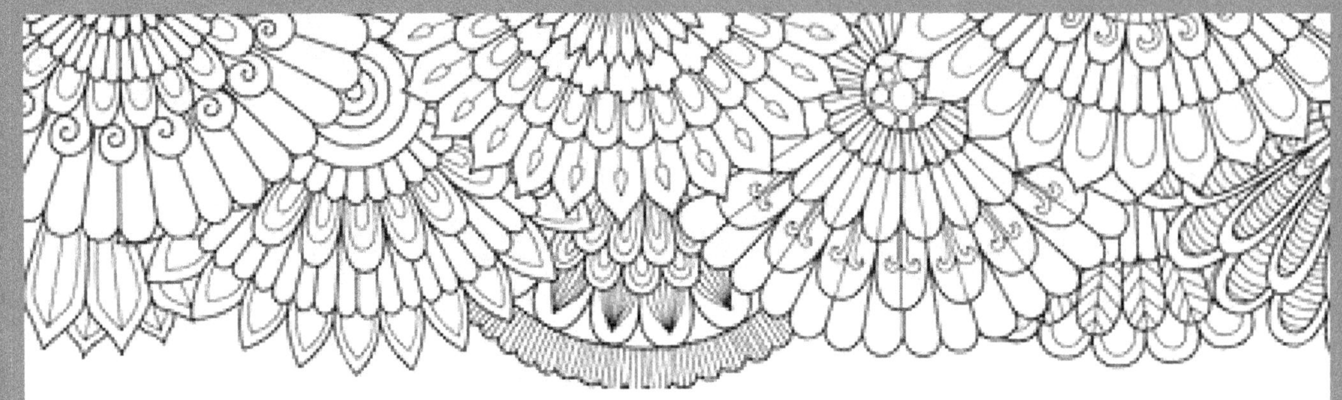

# COW POSE

Cow Pose (Bitilasana) is an easy, gentle way to warm up the spine. It is often paired with Cat Pose (Marjaryasana) for a gentle warm-up sequence. When practiced together, the poses help to stretch the body and prepare it for other activity.

The benefits of this synchronized breath movement will also help you relax and ease some of the day's stress. Flexing and extending the spine can help improve circulation in the discs in your back. It's a basic motion, but one that can be enormously beneficial in supporting the back and easing pain and maintaining a healthy spine, especially if you spend a lot of time sitting.

Bringing movement and flexibility to your spine helps your body to become more coordinated. Include this in your morning routine. You may notice yourself walking taller throughout the day!

"Yoga teaches us to cure what need not be endured and endure what cannot be cured" — **B.K.S Iyengar**

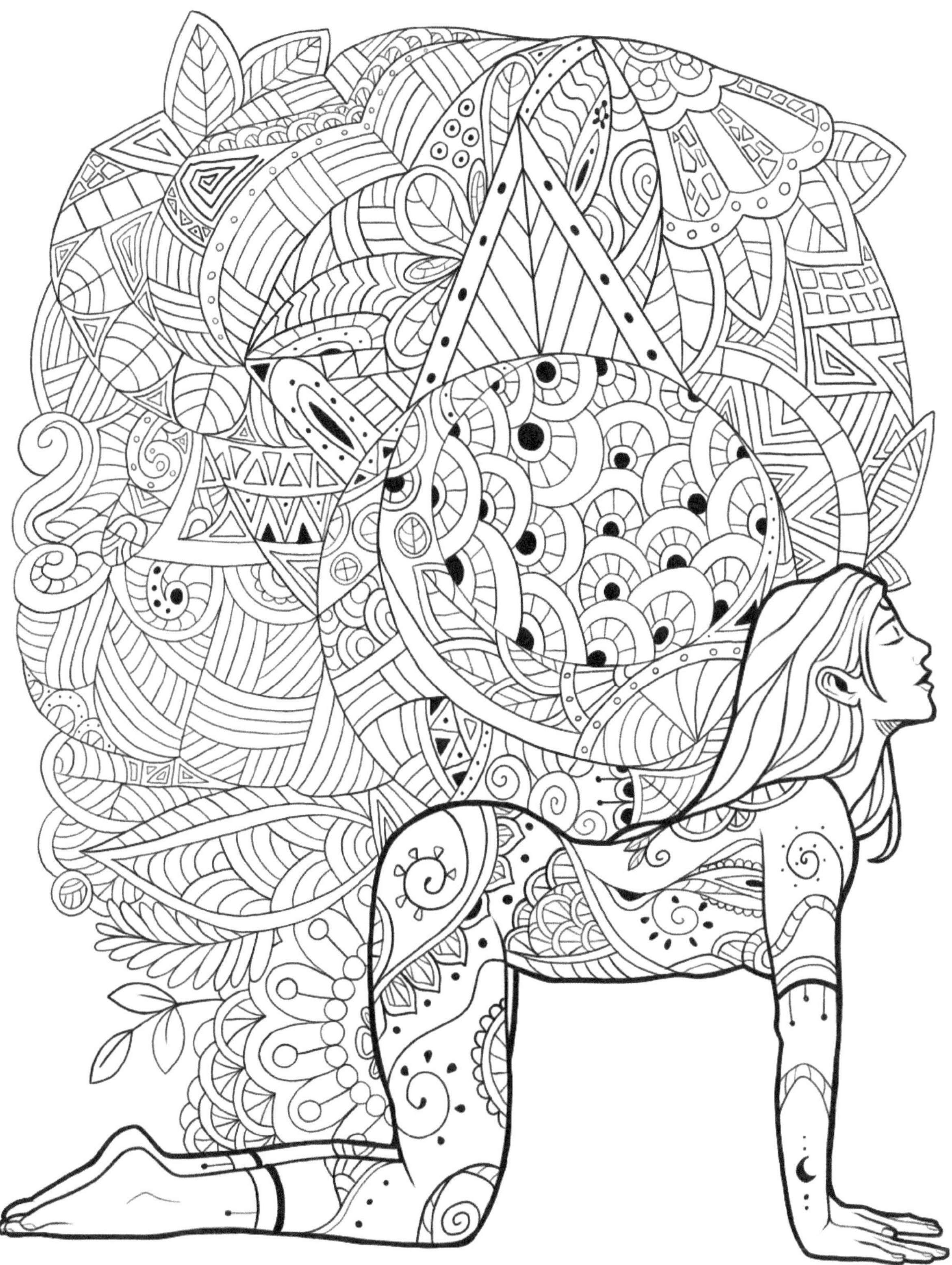

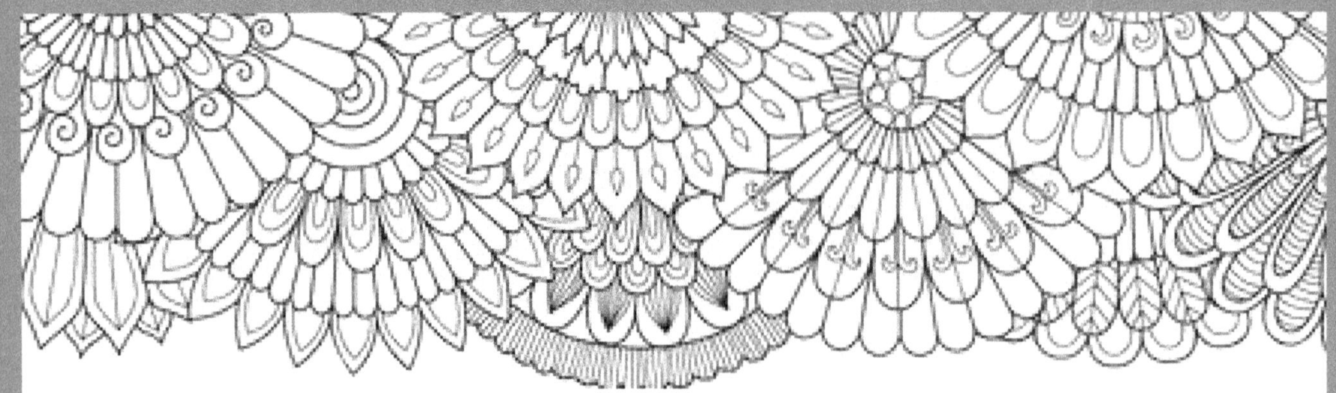

# REVERSIBLE TABLE TOP POSE

Reverse tabletop pose (Ardha Purvottanasana), sometimes called crab pose, opens the chest and tones the low back to stimulate the respiratory and endocrine systems. Reverse tabletop pose also builds arm, leg and core body strength.

This is a yoga posture that stretches the front side of the body and strengthens the core and arm muscles. It is a great pose to counteract a long day of forward-facing action, such as computer work, driving, and traveling. Reverse Table also restores balance to the body after sports and activities that require forward motion, such as swimming, biking, or playing tennis.

Reverse Table can be a useful pose to counteract the forward slouch that results from sitting and forward-facing actions. Regularly practicing Reverse Table can help you stand tall all day long!

"Calming the mind is yoga. Not just standing on the head."
— **Swami Satchidananda**

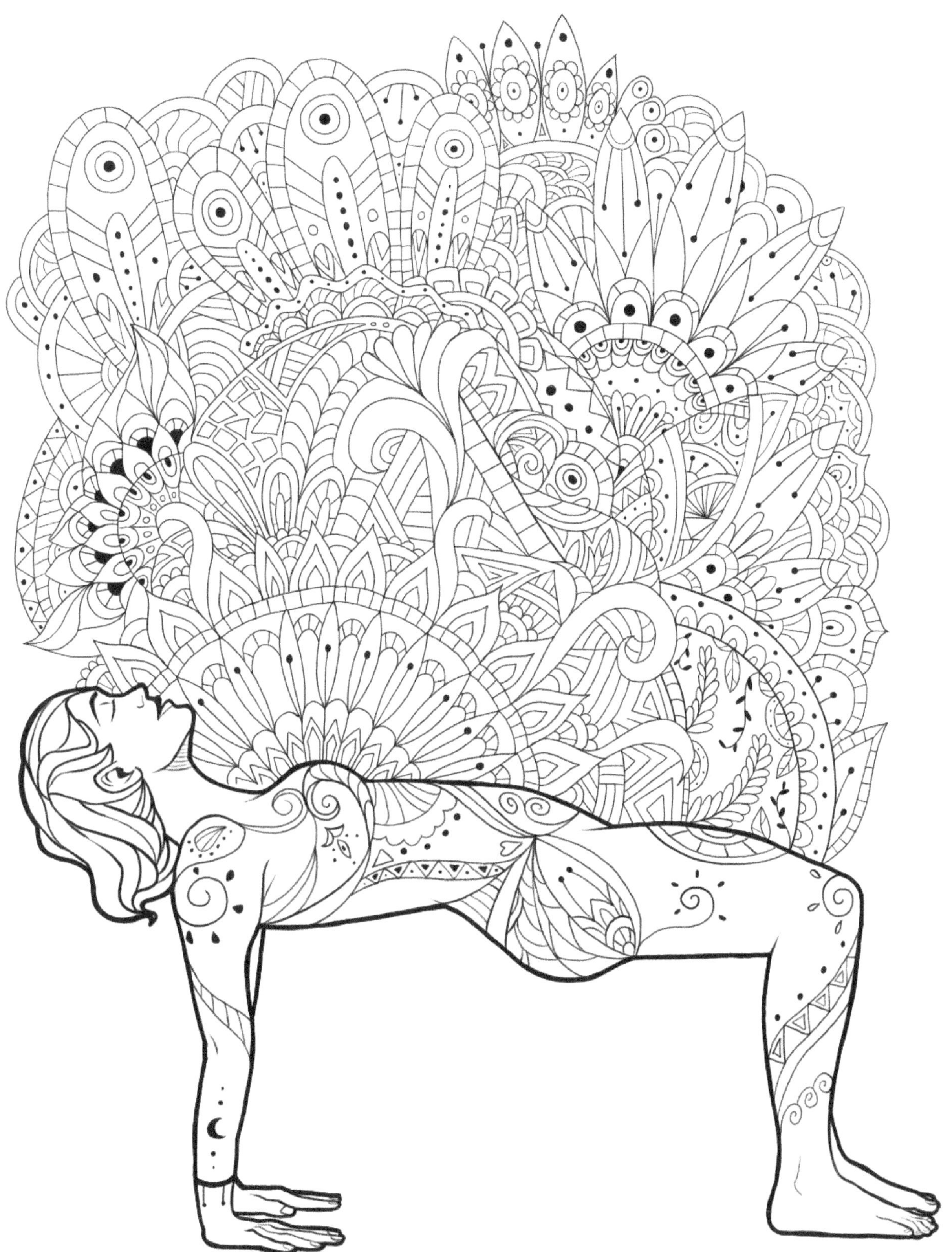

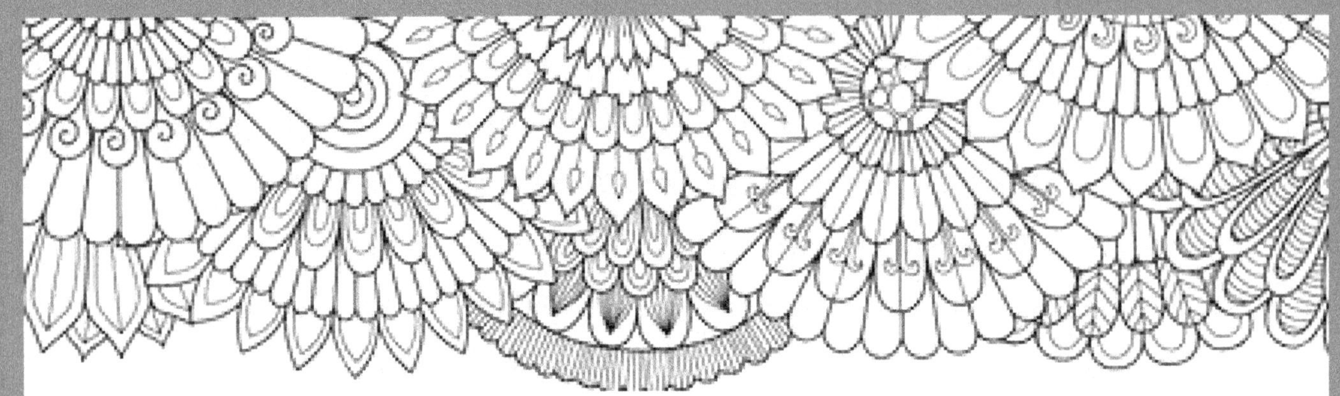

# PLANK POSE

Plank Pose (Kumbhakasana) is an arm balancing yoga pose that tones the abdominal muscles while strengthening the arms and spine.

Practicing Plank Pose for several minutes builds endurance and stamina, while toning the nervous system. The plank is an excellent abdominal and core exercise. It works not only the rectus abdominis, but also the other ab muscles and the core muscles that run from the pelvis along the spine and up to the shoulder girdle.

Nurture your love-hate relationship with Plank Pose. A beginner's best friend, it's the perfect precursor to more challenging arm balances.

"The body is your temple.
Keep it pure and clean for the soul to reside in."
— B.K.S Iyengar

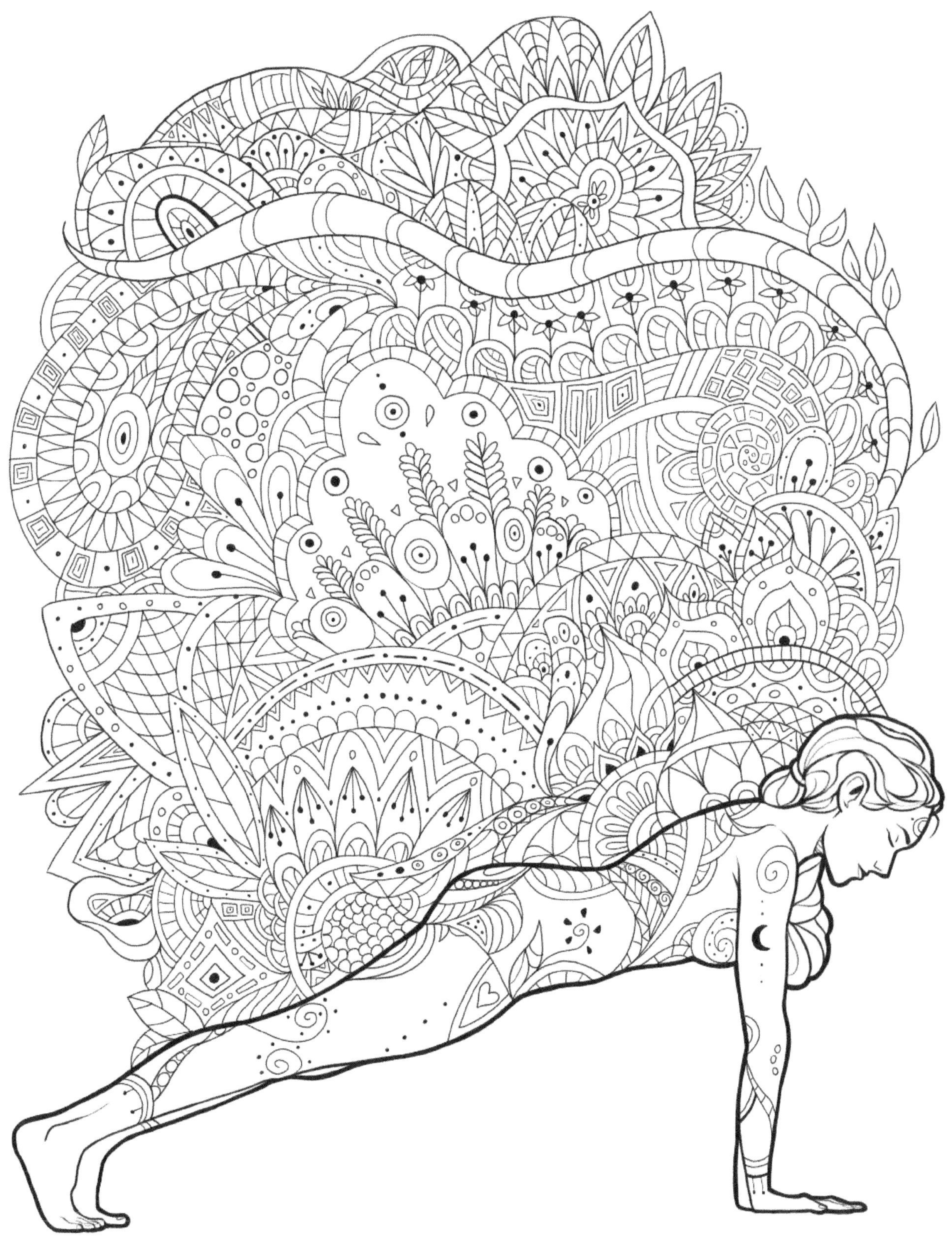

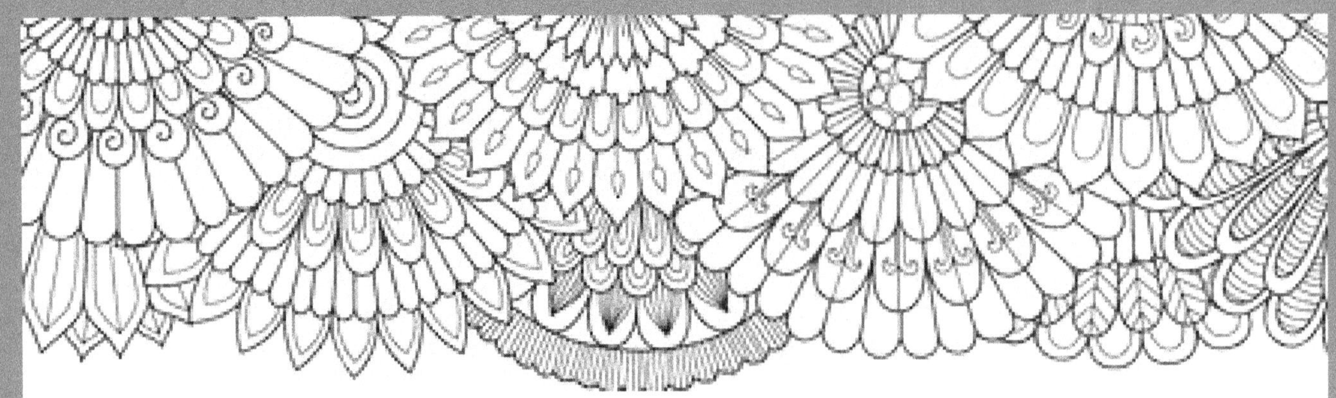

# SIDE PLANK POSE

A powerful arm balance, Side Plank Pose (Vasisthasana) challenges your ability to stay calm and focused.

Vasisthasana strengthens your wrists, forearms, shoulders, and spine. It increases flexibility in the wrists and opens the hips and hamstrings.

It's important to remember that yoga poses can't be conquered or forced. Instead of using sheer muscular effort in the pose, bring your thoughts to your breath and to the power of the present moment. Release your need to achieve a certain outcome and simply be in the now. Stay present with the challenge. The essence of yoga will be revealed to you when you can discover calmness, grace, and ease even in the most physically difficult poses.

"Yoga means addition. Addition of energy, strength and beauty to body, mind and soul." — **Amit Ray**

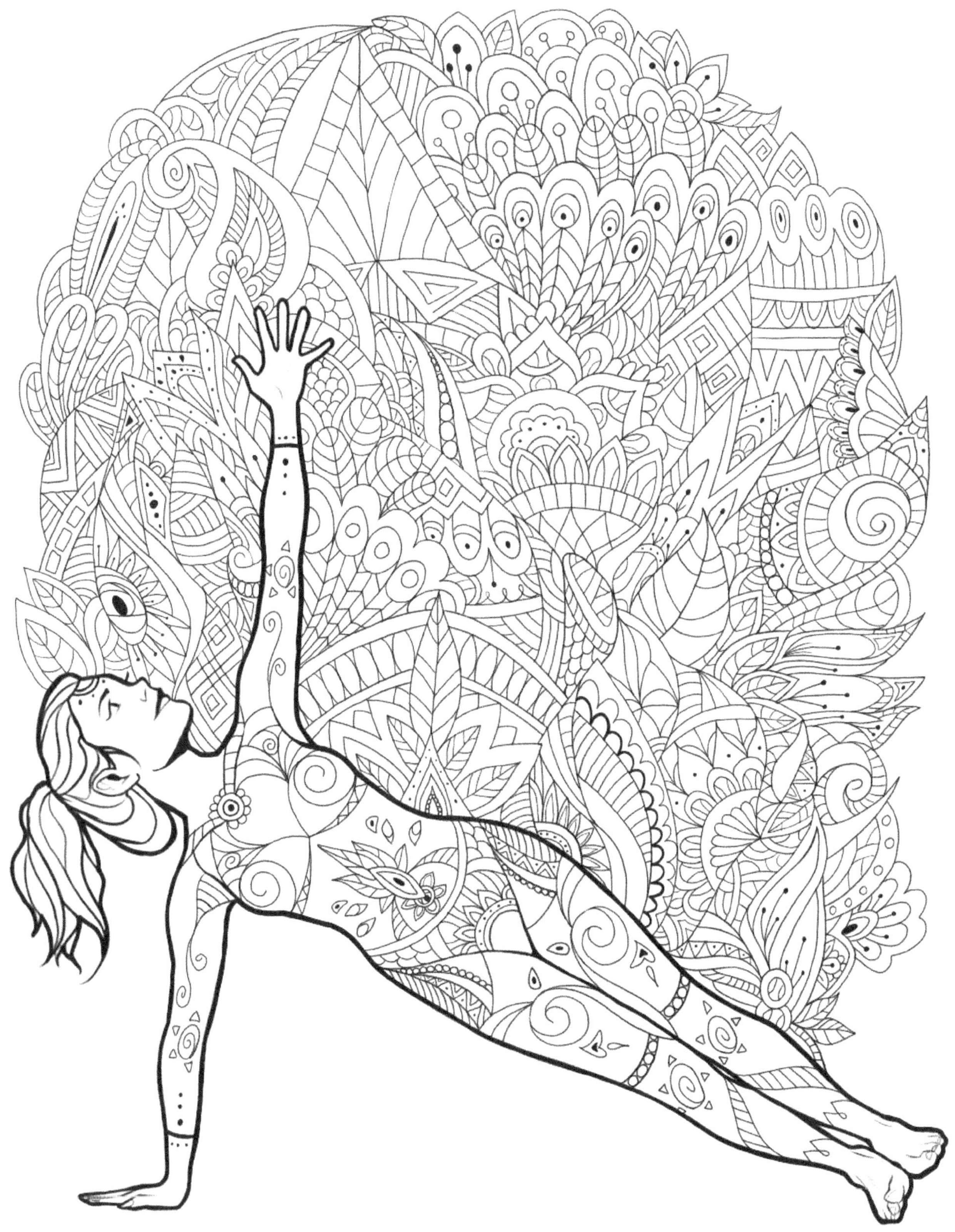

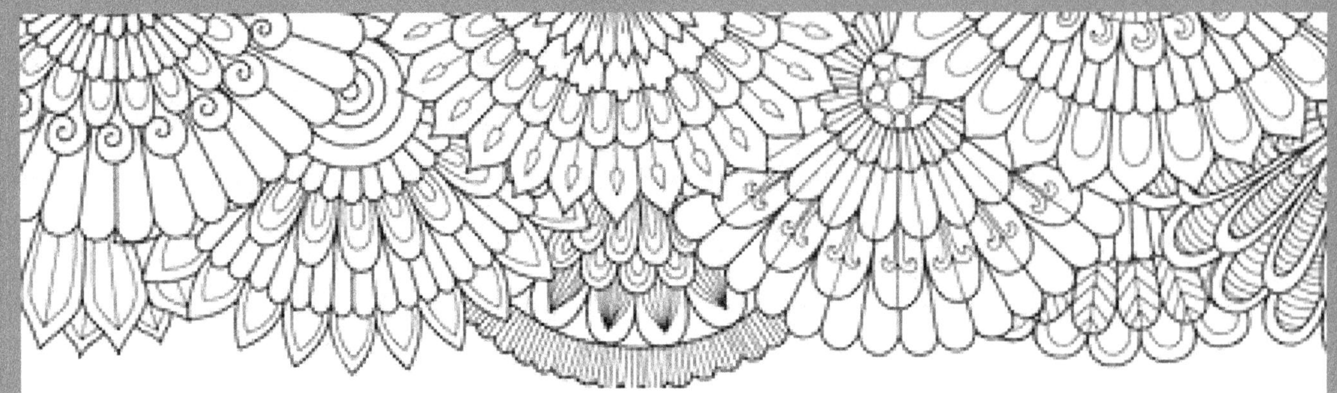

# WARRIOR I POSE

Warrior I (Virabhadrasana I) is a standing yoga pose named after a mythological Hindu warrior, Virabhadra. Warrior I transforms the intensity of this deity into a pose that builds focus, power, and stability.

Regular practice of Warrior I/Virabhadrasana I increases flexibility in the hips and strengthens and tones the legs, ankles and feet. Working on Warrior I will improve all standing poses as well as hip openers. In this pose we get a twist for the spine, while the opening of the shoulders and side body prepares us for backbends.

Warrior I can be a powerful way to build concentration, balance, and focus. It creates strength in all areas of life — physical, mental, emotional, and spiritual. Practicing this pose regularly will help you to face the challenges of daily life with equanimity and poise.

"The very heart of yoga practice is 'abhyasa' steady effort in the direction you want to go." — **Sally Kempton**

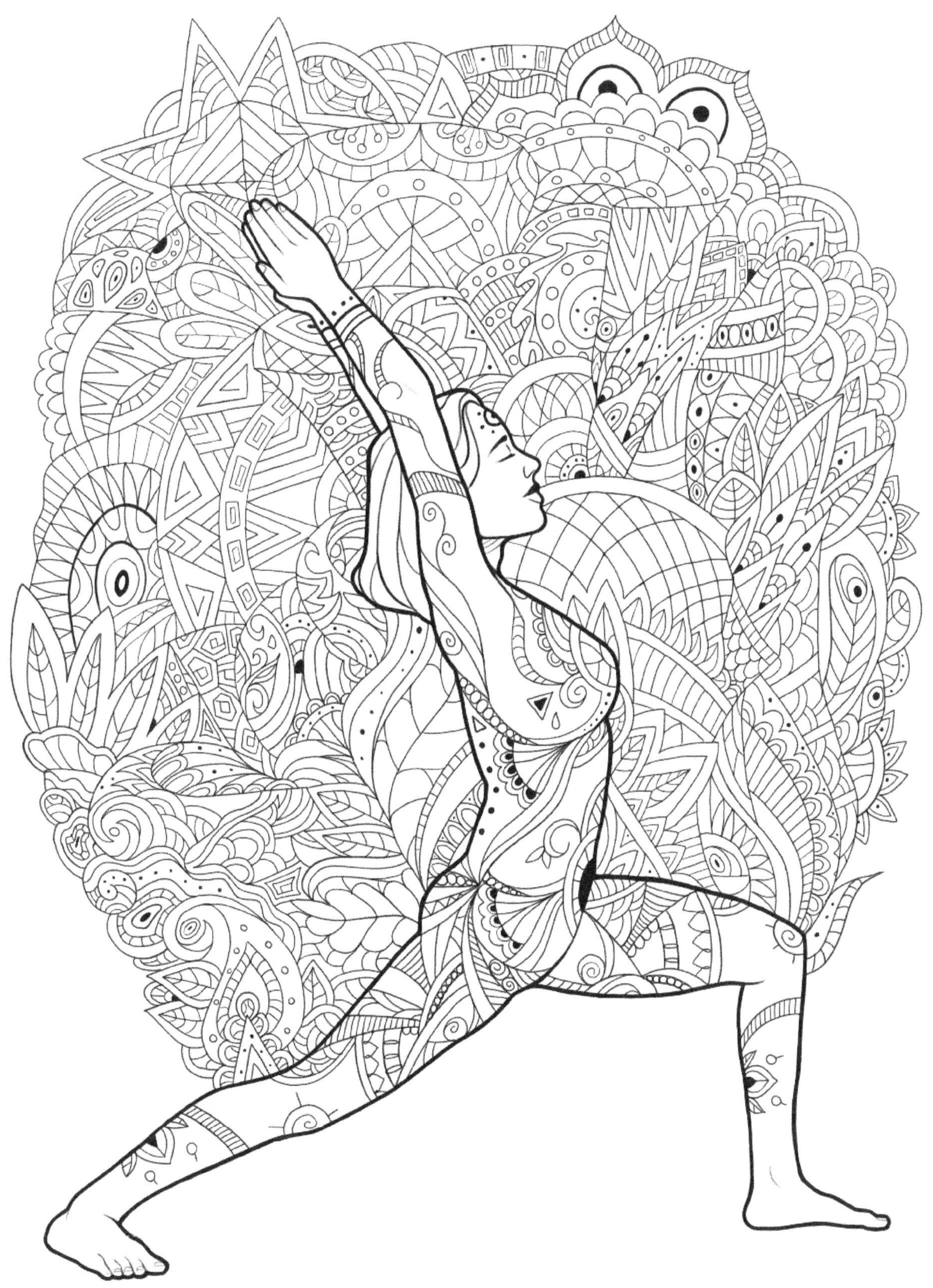

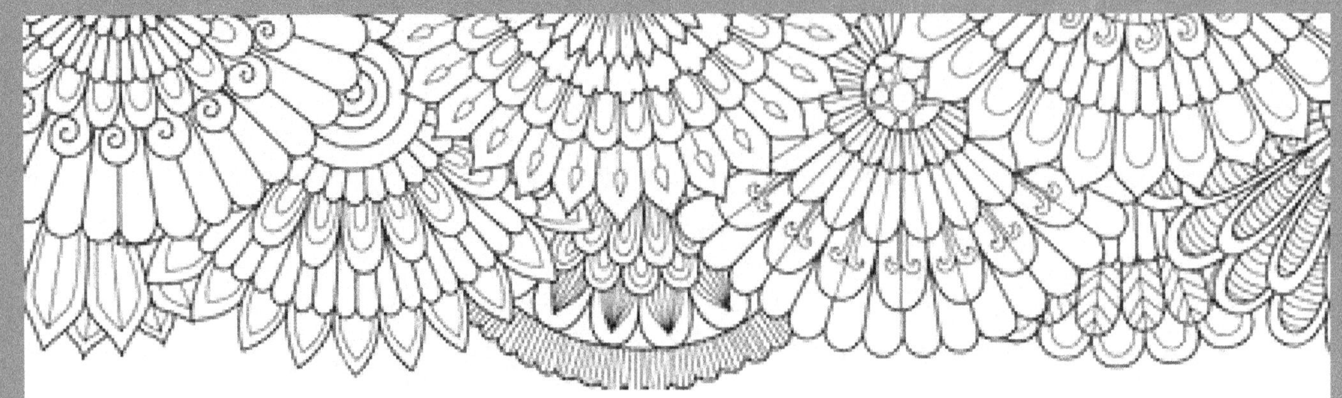

# WARRIOR II POSE

Warrior II (Virabhadrasana II) is a standing yoga pose that enhances strength, stability, and concentration. It's named after the Hindu mythological warrior, Virabhadra, an incarnation of the god Shiva.

Warrior II strengthens the legs, opens the hips and chest. Warrior II develops concentration, balance and groundedness. This pose improves circulation and respiration and energizes the entire body.

Warrior II can be an effective way to build a feeling of inner strength and power. As you practice this pose on a regular basis, you will grow in your ability to face daily battles with ease and grace.

"Yoga is not just repetition of few postures, it is more about the exploration and discovery of the subtle energies of life."
— **Amit Ray**

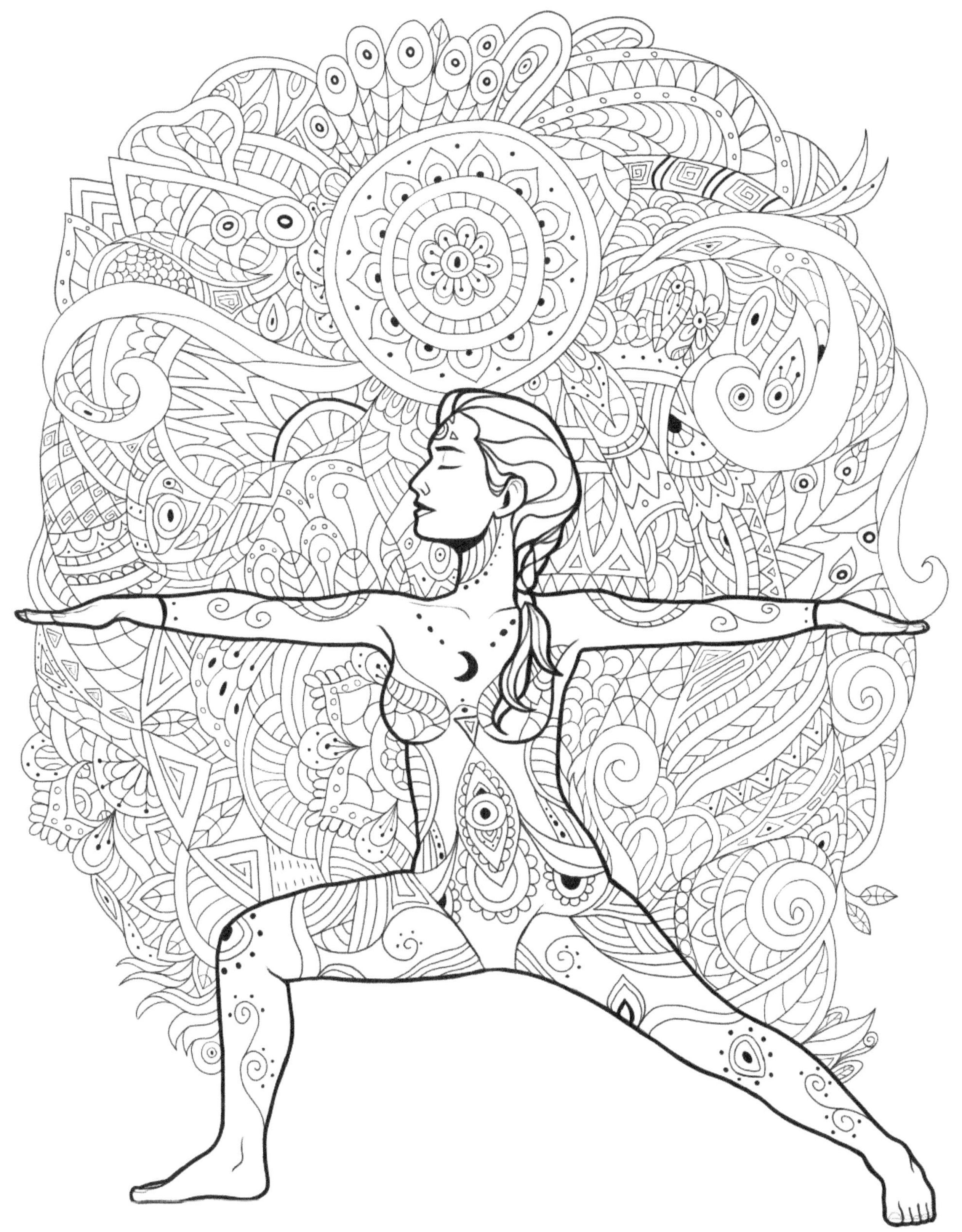

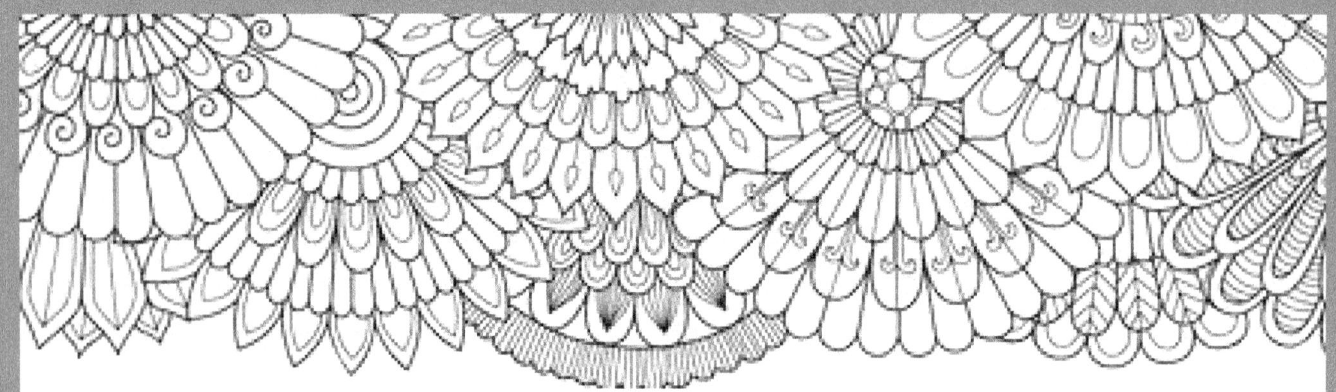

# WARRIOR III POSE

Warrior III (Virabhadrasana III) is an intermediate balancing pose in yoga. This dynamic standing posture creates stability throughout your entire body by integrating all of the muscles throughout your core, arms, and legs.

This pose strengthens the ankles and legs, the shoulders and muscles of the back, tones the abdomen and improves balance and postures.

Practicing Warrior III can be challenging and rewarding on many levels. With patience and dedication, you may discover your ability to face all challenges in life with grace and poise.

"The gift of learning to meditate is the greatest gift
you can give yourself in this lifetime." — **Sogyal Rinpoche**

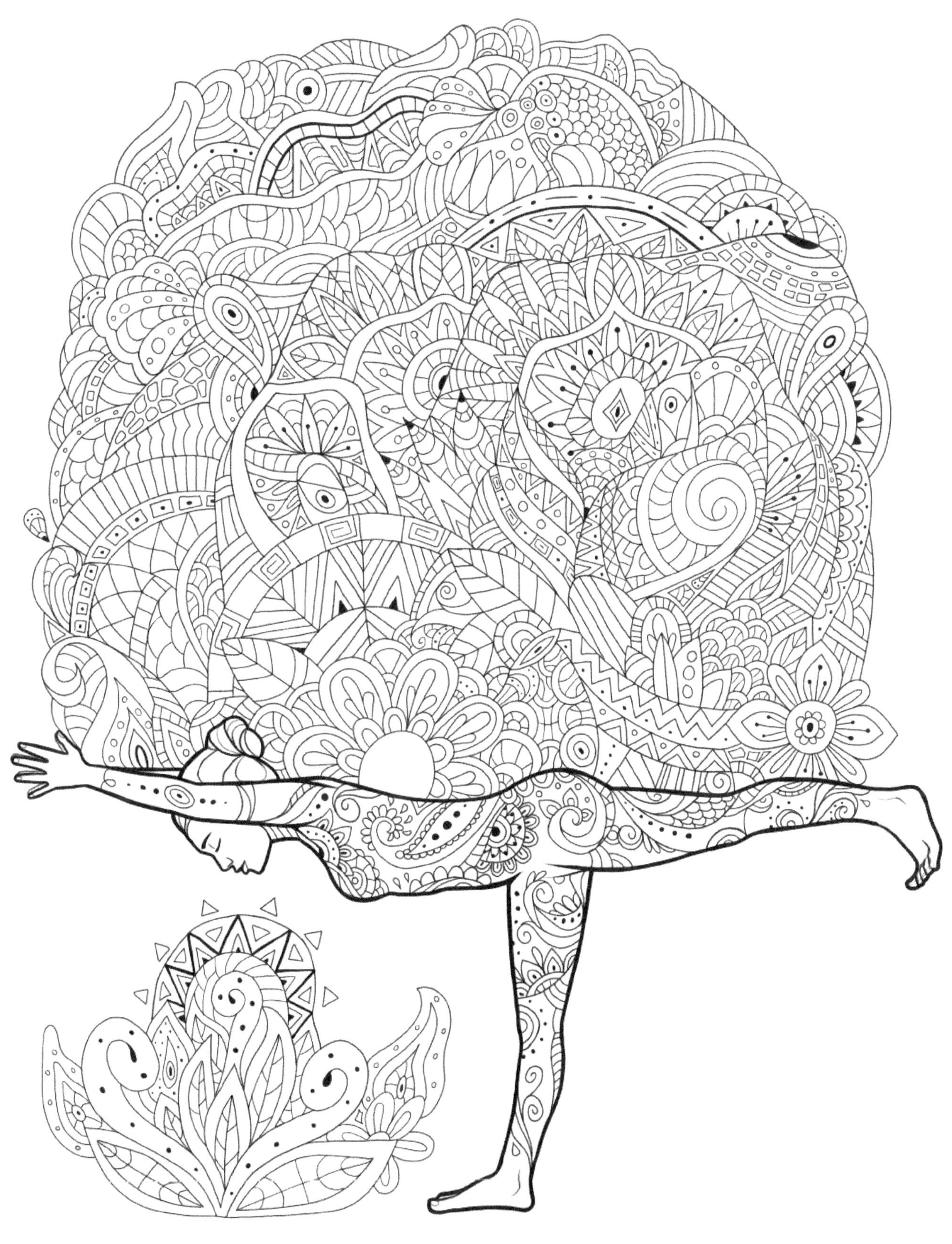

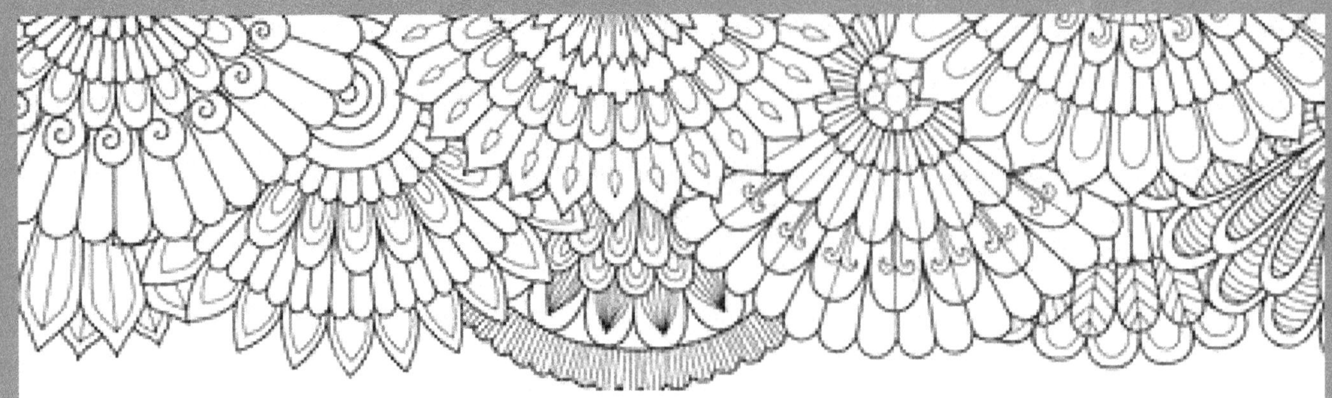

# EXTEND HAND-TO-BIG-TOE POSE

Standing Hand to Big Toe Pose (Utthita Hasta Padangusthasana) is an intermediate yoga posture that stretches the backs of your legs while challenging your balance.

This pose challenges and improves your sense of balance, which in turn develops greater concentration and focus.

This powerful pose will provide your practice with a mental and physical challenge. Remember to take it slowly, and be sure to modify the pose as needed. With practice, your flexibility and your ability to balance will improve.

"Meditation can help us embrace our worries, our fear, our anger; and that is very healing. We let our own natural capacity of healing do the work." — **Thich Nhat Hanh**

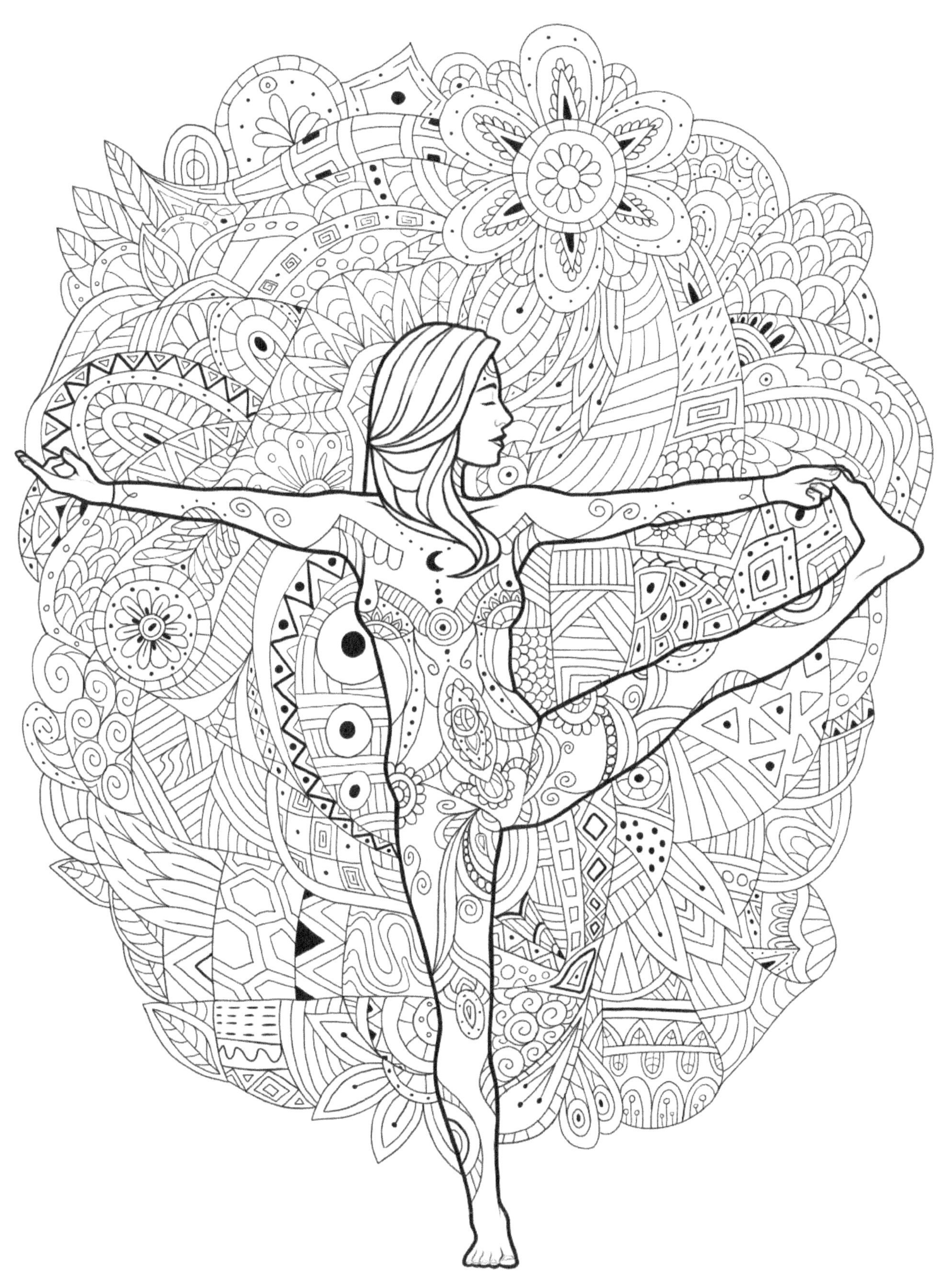

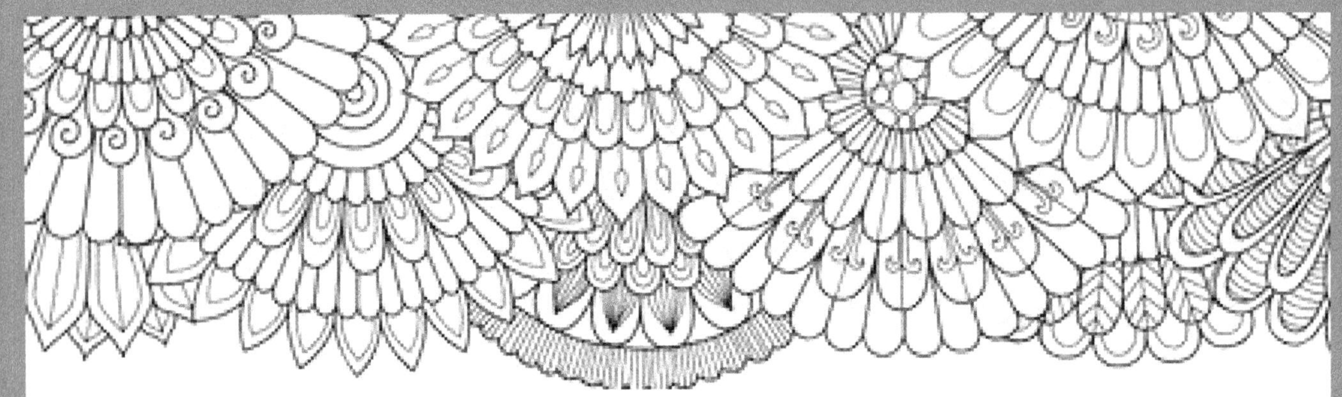

# TREE POSE

Tree Pose (Vrksasana) improves focus and concentration while calming your mind. This strengthens your legs and core while opening your hips and stretching your inner thighs and groin muscles. Also, this pose establishes strength and balance in the legs, and helps you feel centered, steady, and grounded.

Tree Pose connects you to the earth, as you root down through your standing foot. As you balance in the pose, feel the slight and gentle sway of your body.

"Inner peace begins the moment you choose not to allow another person or event to control your emotions."
— **Kathryn Budig**

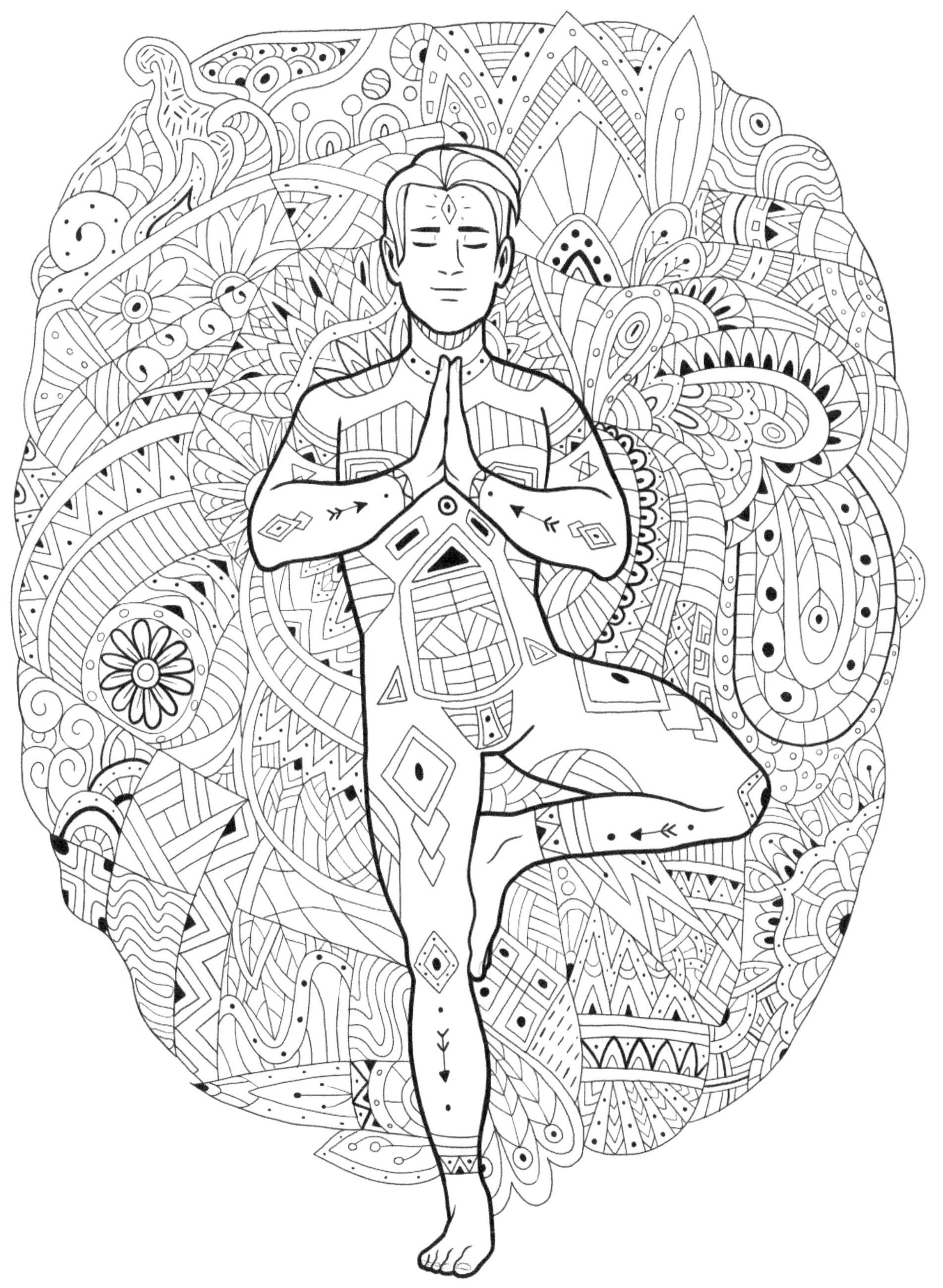

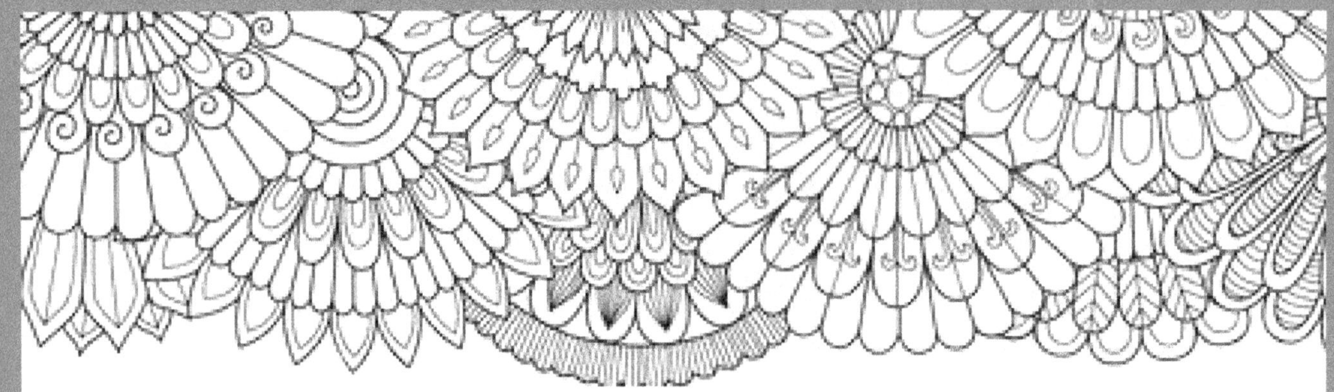

# SUPPORTED HEADSTAND POSE

Standing on your head in proper alignment not only strengthens the whole body but calms the brain.

Inversions, including headstands, may be best known for the simple benefit of getting the heart above the head. When we invert ourselves or go upside down, our blood is given the chance to reverse throughout the body. Also, this pose helps relieve stress, strengthen the spine and upper body, stimulate the pineal gland, helps with insomnia, and improves digestion.

"Your body exists in the past and your mind exists in the future.
In yoga, they come together in the present." — **B.K.S.Iyengar**

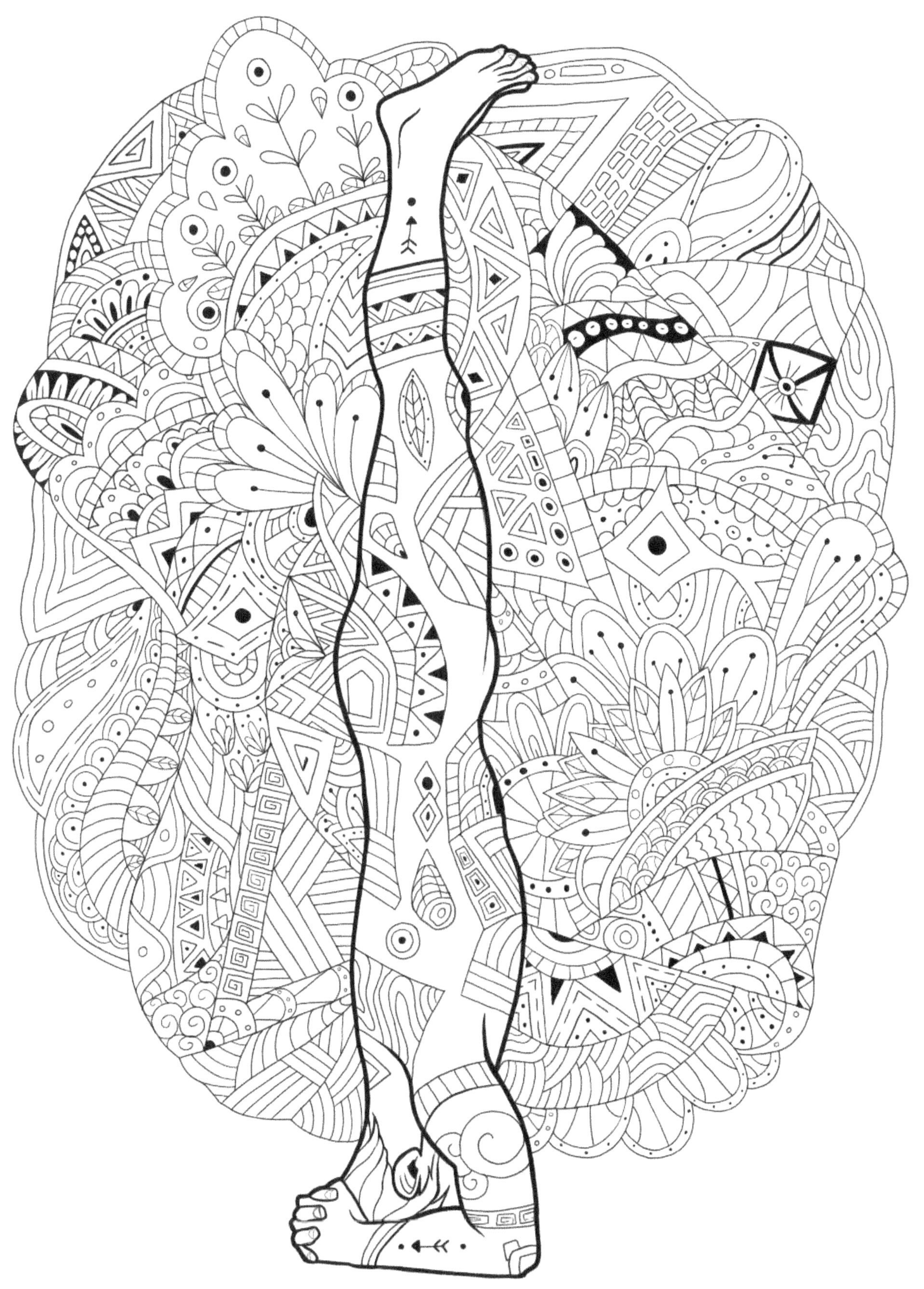

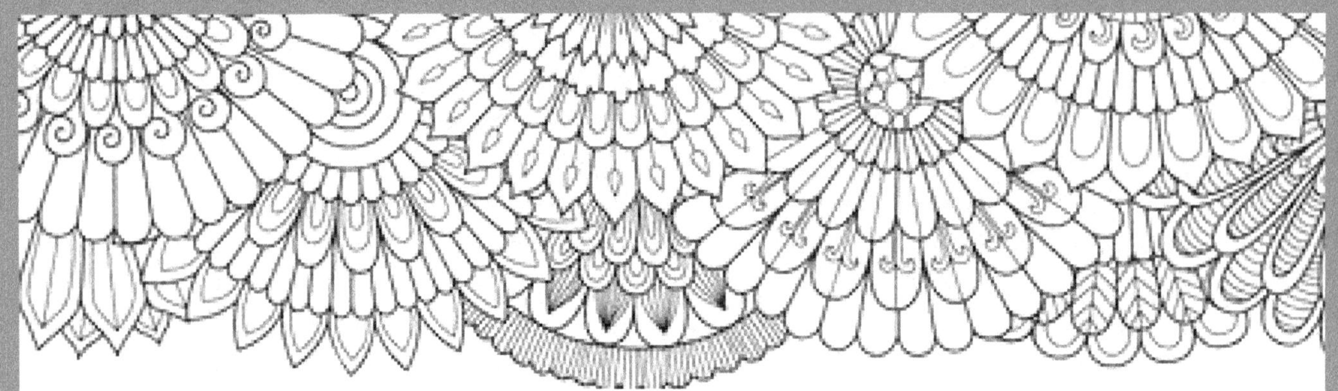

# SCORPION POSE

Scorpion Pose (Vrschikasana) is an advanced-level, backbend pose that uses the entire body's strength to get upside down while balancing on your forearms.

The Scorpion Pose stretches and strengthens all at once. This pose works on shoulders, arms, core, and back. It improves the flexibility of your spine and stretches your hip flexors and chest muscles.

Scorpion Pose can push your limits when it comes to fear and vulnerability while working on your balance and concentration.

"The attitude of gratitude is the highest yoga."
— **Yogi Bhajan**

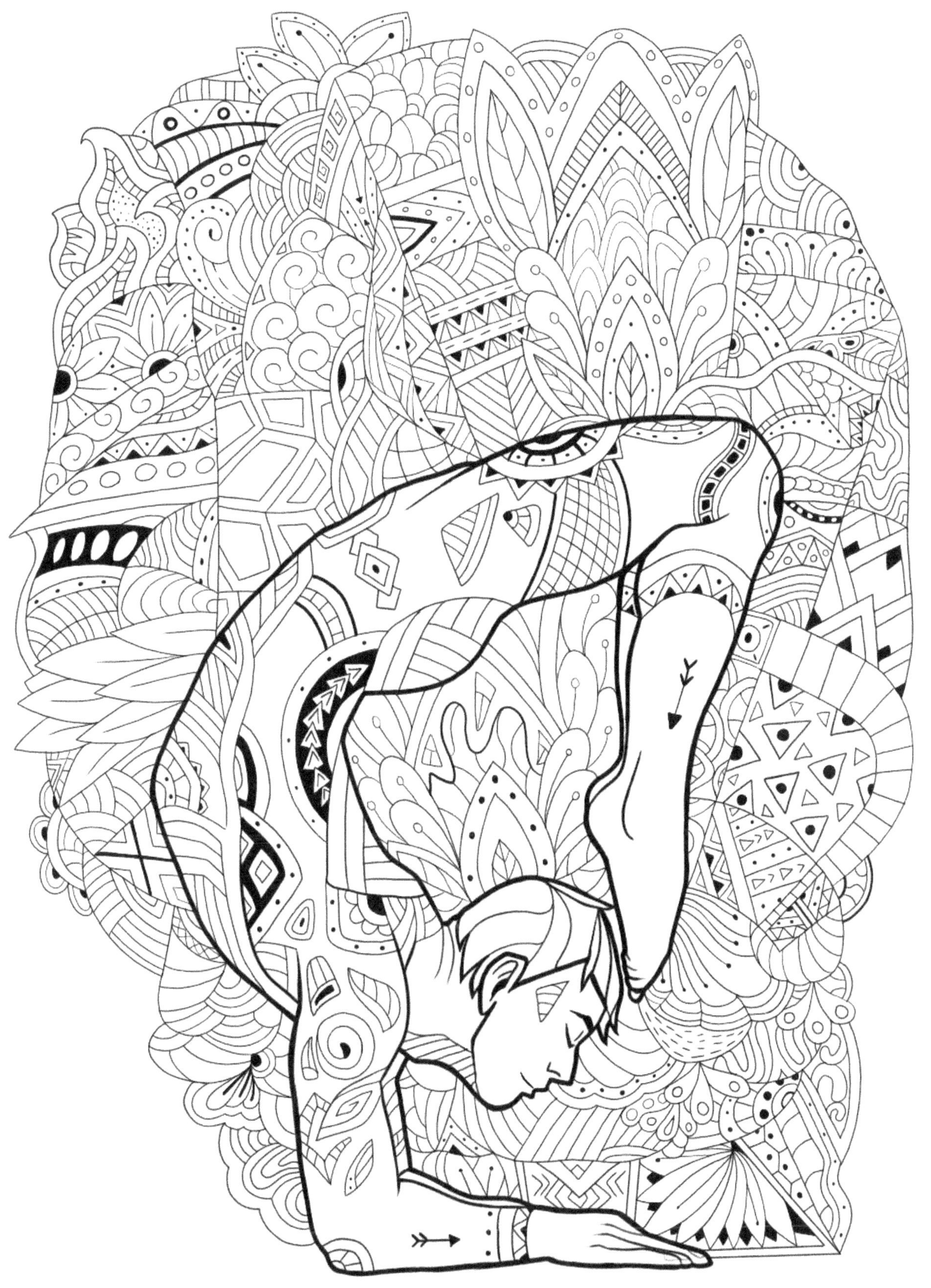

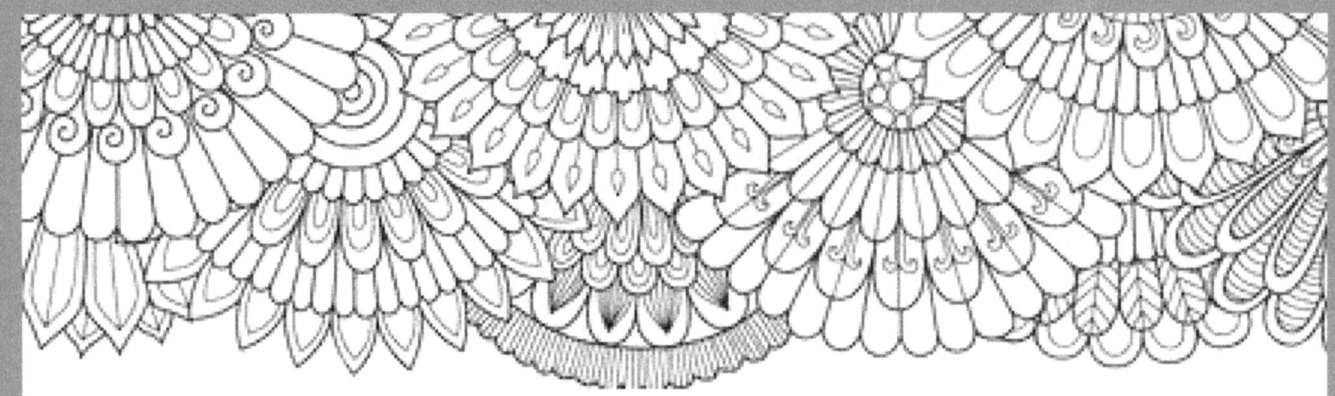

# BIRD OF PARADISE POSE

Bird of Paradise Pose (Svarga Dvijasana) is compared to the real living soul where one needs to work hard on the spiritual front to attain the Heavenly world. Furthermore, this pose requires one to have an immense sense of control and balance not only on the body but from within to remain calm while in the posture.

This pose is a challenging balance that incorporates hip opening, core and back strengthening, and hamstring lengthening.

"Yoga is a method to come to a non dreaming mind.
Yoga is the science to be in the here and now." — **Osho**

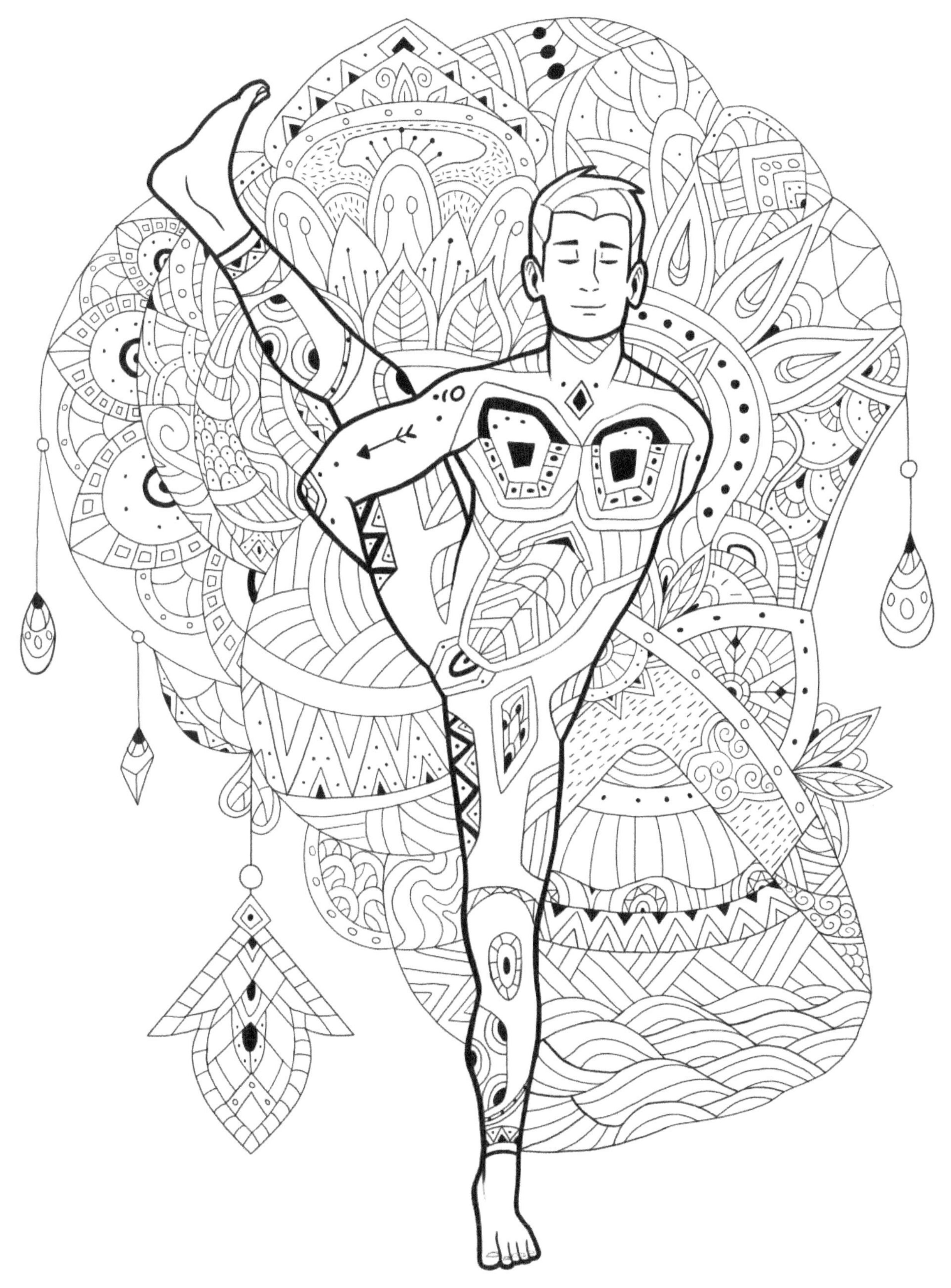

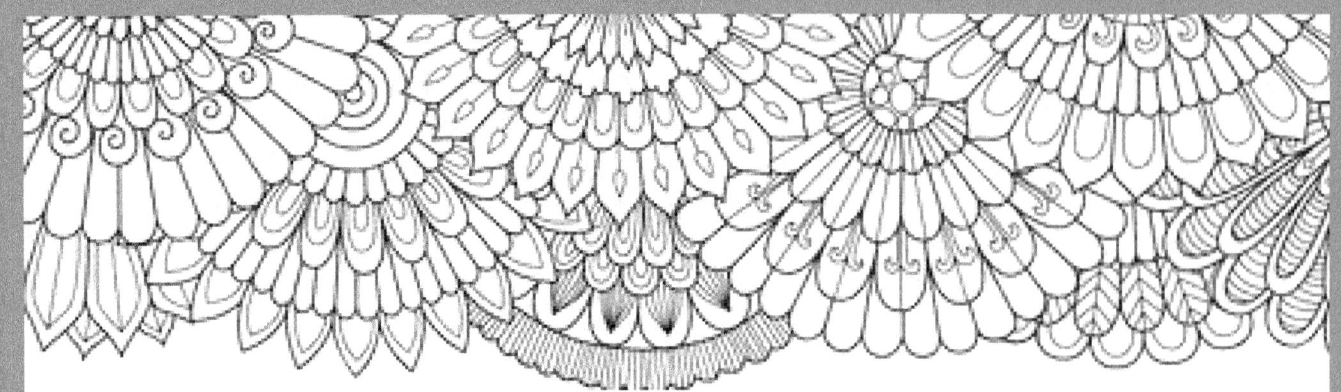

# WILD THING POSE

Wild Thing (Camatkarasana) is an asana that has many names: Rock Star and Flip Dog. This is a pretty good description of the strong back-bending yoga pose, since the open chest does not only open your heart, it also gives you strength and confidence. Thus, this makes it a very powerful yoga pose.

Wild Thing is a yoga pose that stretches the entire front body. This means that it opens up the chest and shoulder area and, thus, creates space in the heart and lungs, boosting the lungs' performance.

"The rhythm of the body, the melody of the mind and the harmony of the soul create the symphony of life."
— B.K.S. Iyengar

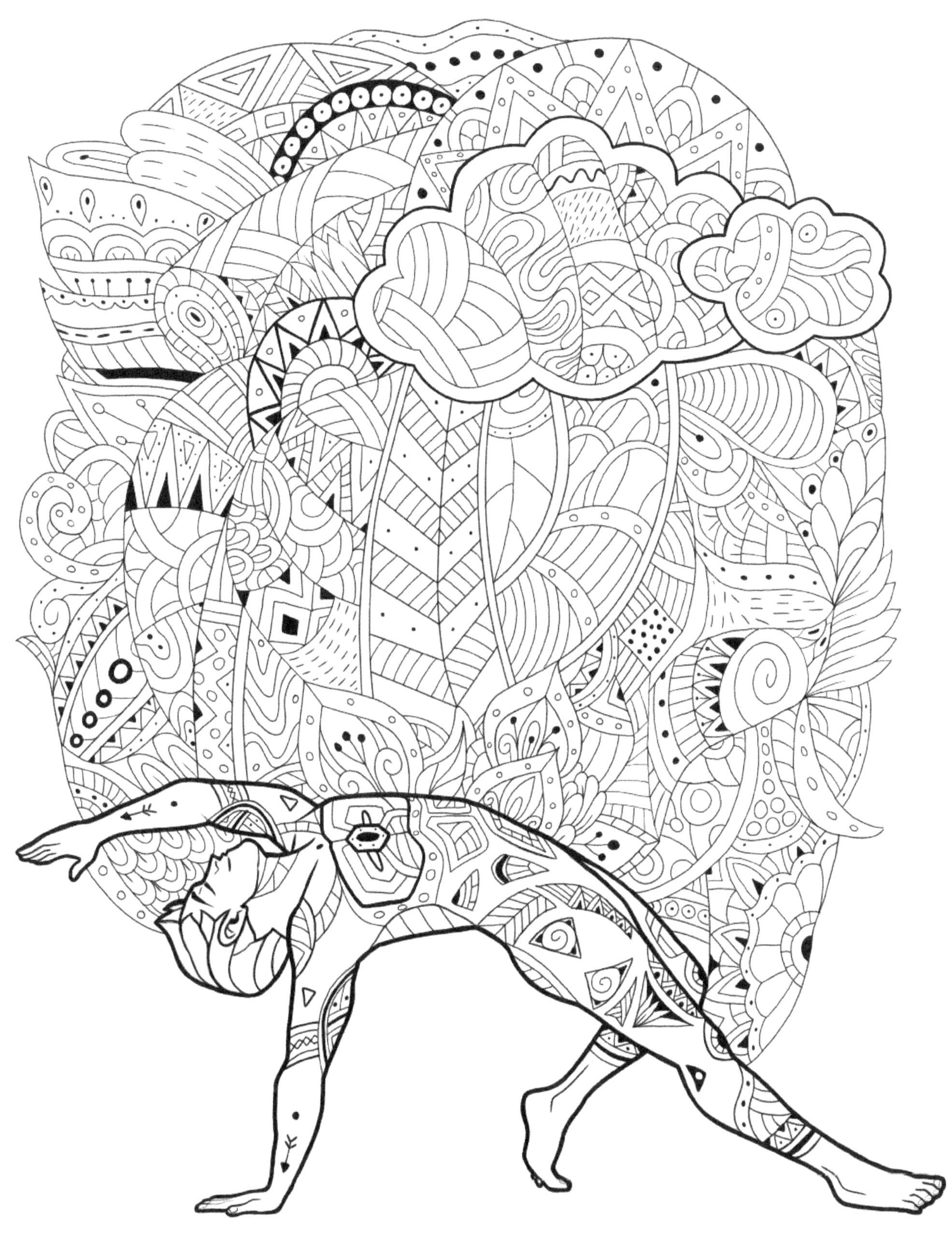

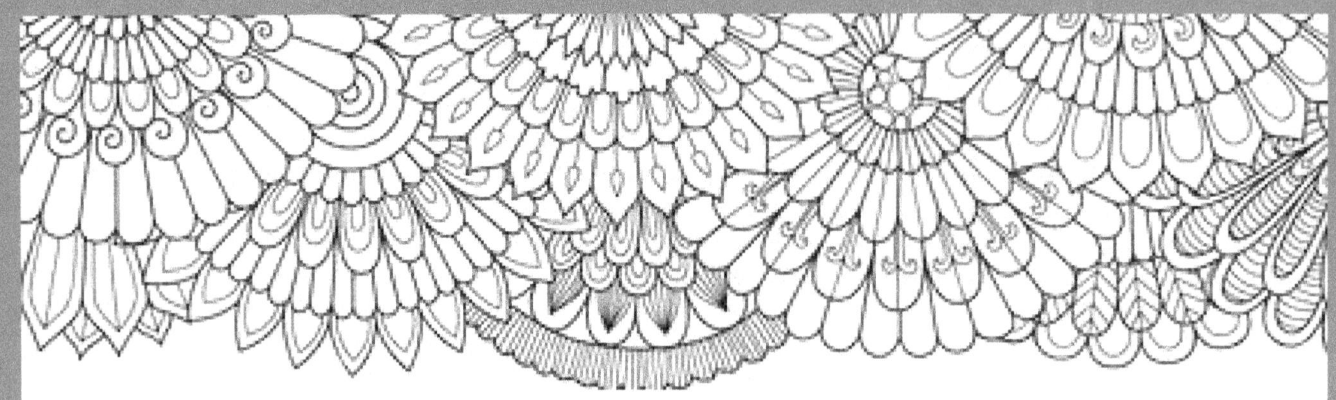

# DON'T FORGET TO LEAVE AN AMAZON REVIEW!

Congratulations on completing this coloring book. We hope we helped you remember your poses while having fun through the beautiful illustrations we had prepared for you. Yoga Coloring Book with Mandala Background was created to give you hours of relaxation, motivation, and new learning while unleashing the creativity in you!

Continue doing your poses every day, and we'll see you on your next yoga coloring journey! Namaste!

If you liked this book, then we'd appreciate you letting us know through an honest review in the Amazon product page. Reviews are the lifeblood of our publishing endeavors. A 5-star review would mean the world to us. We're counting with yours!

Thank you for choosing **Dreamstorm Publications.**

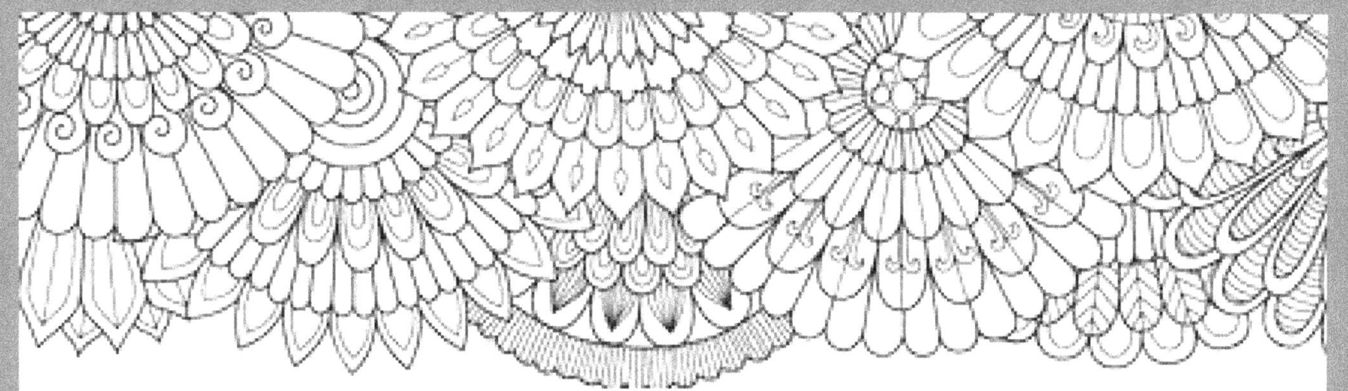

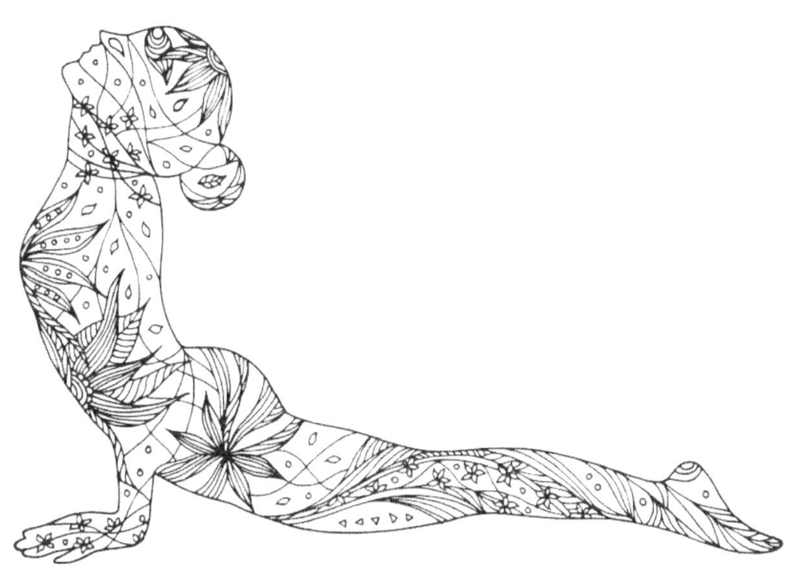

When you cannot control what is happening,
challenge yourself to control the way you respond
to what is happening. That's where your power is.